NANCY EVE THOMAS, M.D., F.A.C.S.
4801 Massachusetts Avenue, N.W.
Washington, D.C. 20016
363-4300

Current concepts of the vitreous

including vitrectomy

Current concepts of the vitreous

including vitrectomy

Edited by

Kurt A. Gitter, M.D., F.A.C.S.

Director, Eye Research Laboratory, Touro Infirmary;
Consultant, United States Public Health Service Hospital,
New Orleans, Louisiana

with 271 illustrations

The C. V. Mosby Company

Saint Louis   1976

Library of Congress Cataloging in Publication Data

Main entry under title:

Current concepts of the vitreous including vitrectomy.

    Proceedings of a tutorial conference held in
April 1975 in New Orleans, sponsored by Touro Infirmary
Eye Research Laboratory.
    Includes bibliographical references and index.
    1. Vitreous body—Surgery—Congresses.
I. Gitter, Kurt A., 1937-   [DNLM: 1. Vitreous
body—Congresses. 2. Vitreous body—Surgery—Congresses.
WW250 C976 1975]
RE80.C87   617.7'46   75-37985
ISBN 0-8016-1845-2

VH/VH/VH 9 8 7 6 5 4 3 2 1

Contributors

Gerald Cohen, M.D.

Eye Research Laboratory, Touro Infirmary; Consultant, United States
Public Health Service Hospital, New Orleans, Louisiana

D. Jackson Coleman, M.D.

Assistant Professor of Clinical Ophthalmology, Department of
Ophthalmology, College of Physicians and Surgeons of
Columbia University, New York, New York

Nicholas G. Douvas, M.D.

Director, Port Huron Eye Clinic, Port Huron, Michigan

Kurt A. Gitter, M.D.

Director, Eye Research Laboratory, Touro Infirmary; Consultant,
United States Public Health Service Hospital,
New Orleans, Louisiana

Morton F. Goldberg, M.D.

Professor and Head, Department of Ophthalmology, Eye and Ear Infirmary,
University of Illinois Hospital, Chicago, Illinois

Felipe U. Huamonte, M.D.

Department of Ophthalmology, Eye and Ear Infirmary,
University of Illinois Hospital, Chicago, Illinois

Norman S. Jaffe, M.D.

Clinical Professor of Ophthalmology, Bascom Palmer Eye Institute,
University of Miami, School of Medicine, Miami, Florida

David Kasner, M.D.

Clinical Professor of Ophthalmology, Bascom Palmer Eye Institute,
University of Miami, School of Medicine, Miami, Florida

Ronald G. Michels, M.D.

Assistant Professor of Ophthalmology, Department of Ophthalmology,
The Johns Hopkins University School of Medicine, Baltimore, Maryland

Edward Okun, M.D.

Associate Professor of Clinical Ophthalmology, Department of Ophthalmology,
Washington University School of Medicine, St. Louis, Missouri

Gholam A. Peyman, M.D.

Department of Ophthalmology, Eye and Ear Infirmary,
University of Illinois Hospital, Chicago, Illinois

Stephen J. Ryan, Jr., M.D.

Professor and Chairman, Department of Ophthalmology,
University of Southern California, Los Angeles, California

Jerry A. Shields, M.D.

Senior Assistant Surgeon, Oncology Unit, Retina Service, Wills Eye
Hospital; Assistant Professor of Ophthalmology, Thomas Jefferson
University and Temple University, Philadelphia, Pennsylvania

To

MILLIE, LINDA, GREG, RICK, and DOUG

Preface

New techniques and instrumentation developed for vitreous surgery over the past several years have prompted innovative and exciting therapeutic possibilities.

After attending the University of California Symposium on Vitreous Surgery in March, 1974, I found it apparent that the original pioneering efforts in vitreous surgery had given way to a new era of clinical vitreous surgical capability. Accordingly, I organized a tutorial conference in New Orleans in April, 1975, sponsored by Touro Infirmary Eye Research Laboratory, at which a distinguished faculty was assembled. I am proud to have had the opportunity to work with these astute clinicians and teachers in organizing both the tutorial conference and the contents of this text.

Dr. Jerry Shields provides an outstanding introduction to the symposium with lectures on the normal anatomy of the vitreous and its pathology.

Drs. Nicholas Douvas and Gholam Peyman, both innovative surgeons and pioneers in instrument design, provide insights as to their instrumentation and clinical experience with vitreous surgery.

Dr. Norman Jaffe adds significantly by incorporating his knowledge of anterior chamber surgery with complications of the vitreous.

Drs. Stephen Ryan and Ronald Michels and Dr. Edward Okun share their clinical judgment and experience with vitrectomy in several hundred cases. In addition, Drs. Ryan and Michels elaborate on the proper preoperative evaluation of vitrectomy patients.

Dr. Jackson Coleman elucidates the benefits of ultrasonic diagnosis in the preoperative evaluation of vitrectomy candidates. He also describes his techniques in trauma cases, with which he has had considerable experience.

My associate, Dr. Gerald Cohen, and I present data on complications of vitrectomy in over 385 cases.

Our moderators at the conference included Drs. Walter Cockerham, Gerald Cohen, Gholam Peyman, Mercer McClure, and David Kasner. They acted in multiple capacities by introducing speakers, organizing panel discussions, and providing minilectures. All the moderators were vital to this symposium, but none more than Dr. Kasner, the pioneer of open sky vitrectomy, whose presence was electrifying throughout the 2-day meeting.

The round table impromptu discussions were edited (by me) but do reflect the honest and unobstructed views of the panelists and hopefully will be well received by our readers.

This book is not intended to be the final or ultimate statement on disorders and surgery of the vitreous but rather a reflection of contemporary thought. Hopefully it will act as a stimulus to further clinical and basic research.

I am indebted in all my academic pursuits to my excellent residency training at Wills Eye Hospital under Dr. Arthur Keeney, my friend and mentor. The Retina Service at Wills promoted my initial interest in the posterior segment, which has not dampened over the years.

I would particularly like to thank Touro Infirmary Hospital and its board for its commitment in establishing and maintaining our eye research laboratory. I am indebted to the many individuals, groups, and pharmaceutical companies who over the past six years have generously aided our clinical research efforts and our annual ophthalmic symposium. Most important among them has been Jack Aron. I would like to thank my entire office staff and the public relations department of Touro Infirmary, without whose efforts this symposium would have been impossible.

Finally, I thank my wife, Millie, and my four children, Linda Leigh, Gregory, Richard, and Douglas, for their kindness and understanding in sharing these times with me.

Kurt A. Gitter

Contents

Current concepts of the vitreous

including vitrectomy

1

Surgical anatomy of the vitreous

JERRY A. SHIELDS

For both the ophthalmologist and the ophthalmic pathologist the vitreous is one of the most difficult structures of the eye to study. Because of its transparency and relative inaccessibility, the ophthalmologist may find it difficult to examine; and since it is 99% water and often lost in routine preparations of eyes, the ophthalmic pathologist also finds it a difficult substance to evaluate.

In recent years ophthalmologists have become increasingly aware that the vitreous plays a significant role in the pathogenesis of a number of disorders involving the adjacent intraocular structures and the eye as a whole. With the realization that the vitreous can be disturbed in vivo without endangering the health of the eye[6] and with the development of specialized surgical instruments for removing or manipulating the vitreous,[9] there has been a recent upsurge of interest in its structure and pathologic reactions.

This chapter will consider the anatomy of the vitreous and its relationship to adjacent structures. Emphasis will be placed on features which are of clinical importance to the ophthalmic surgeon. Only pertinent highlights will be considered here, however; for more details Jaffe's comprehensive textbook is recommended.[5]

GROSS ANATOMY[4,5]

The adult vitreous in the normal state is a transparent gel occupying approximately the posterior two thirds of the globe. It conforms mainly to the structures adjacent to the vitreous cavity—being bounded anteriorly by the lens and zonules, laterally by the ciliary body and peripheral retina, and posteriorly by the retina and optic disc (Fig. 1-1). Anteriorly it has a concave depression, the patellar fossa, which houses the posterior portion of the lens. These anatomic relationships may be best illustrated with a diagram (Fig. 1-2).

Hyaloid membrane

When examined with the slit lamp or dissecting microscope, the vitreous gel appears to be lined by a condensed membrane which conforms to the lens cap-

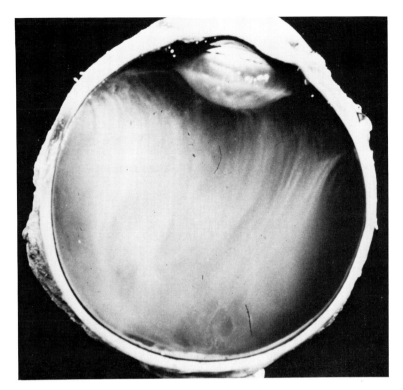

Fig. 1-1. Note that the vitreous in this sectioned eye has turned slightly white in formalin fixation, accentuating its fibrillar structure (AFIP acc. no. 82133).

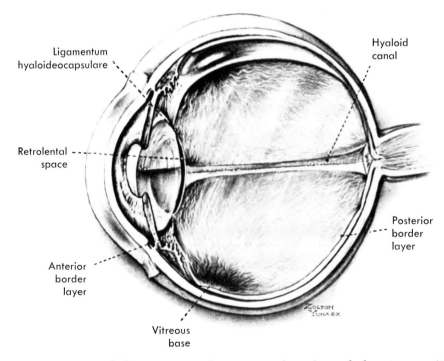

Fig. 1-2. Diagram of the structure and anatomic relationships of the vitreous. (From Hogan, M. J., and Zimmerman, L. E.: Ophthalmic pathology, Philadelphia, 1962, W. B. Saunders Co.)

sule and zonules anteriorly and to the inner surface of the retina posteriorly. With careful biomicroscopy this membrane can be visualized anteriorly; but it is virtually impossible to detect posteriorly unless a posterior vitreous detachment is present. Most authorities believe that it is not a true membrane but rather condensed fibrils of the cortical vitreous. Hence they prefer the terms *anterior border layer* and *posterior border layer*.

The vitreous may be divided into a cortical zone and a central zone, which are difficult to differentiate clinically. The cortical zone, adjacent to the retina, is the more condensed portion; the central, or medullary, vitreous is less condensed and extends from the cortical vitreous centrally to the walls of the hyaloid canal.

Attachments

The degree of adherence of the vitreous gel to adjacent structures varies in different portions of the eye.

The vitreous base, in the region of the peripheral retina and pars plana (Fig. 1-2), is the firmest attachment of the vitreous. It is a ringlike zone of adherence which straddles the ora serrata for 360°, extending from approximately 1 mm posterior to 1.5 mm anterior to the ora and terminating in the

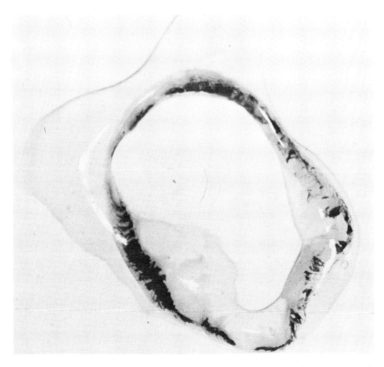

Fig. 1-3. Vitreous gel after removal from an autopsy eye. Note the pigmented ring representing the attachment of the vitreous base to the epithelium of the pars plana.

midportion of the pars plana. The attachment here is so firm that forceful traction on the vitreous in this region will usually detach the pigment epithelium of the pars plana (Fig. 1-3).

More posteriorly the vitreous is less firmly attached to the inner surface of the retina. The attachment here is so tenuous that separation usually occurs when the eye is sectioned in the laboratory. The vitreous gel, however, is somewhat more firmly attached to the margins of the optic disc; but there is no attachment over the central portion of the optic nerve head corresponding to the posterior limit of the hyaloid canal. The vitreous is a little more firmly attached to the macula than to other parts of the retina although there are very few vitreous fibrils in the center of the fovea.

The anterior border layer of the vitreous extends from the anterior limit of the vitreous base centrally to the equatorial region of the lens. It attaches to the posterior surface of the lens periphery, forming a ringlike condensation about 9 mm in diameter known as the hyaloideocapsular ligament, or Weiger's ligament. This attachment is more firm in young people and is believed to account for the frequent loss of vitreous during intracapsular cataract surgery in these patients. Within the ring formed by the hyaloideocapsular ligament is the retrolental space, or Berger's space, which is actually a potential space between the posterior lens capsule and the anterior vitreous that becomes patent only when certain pathologic conditions cause blood or inflammatory cells to collect there.

Passing from the retrolental space to the optic disc is the hyaloid canal, or Cloquet's canal (Fig. 1-2)—an S-shaped tubular structure whose condensed walls represent the only remnants of the primary vitreous in the normal adult eye.

Zonules

The zonules, collectively called the suspensory ligament of the lens, consist of fine fibers passing from the ciliary body to the equatorial region of the lens. Some zonular fibers pass posteriorly across the pars plana, inserting into the dentate processes of the peripheral retina, and producing chronic traction on the peripheral retina. The zonules may have significance in the development of retinal detachments, particularly in aphakic patients.

Relationship of vitreous to pars plana

The pars plana region has become the preferred area for surgically entering the vitreous. The surgeon must remember that the ciliary body extends 6 or 7 mm posterior to the limbus on the temporal side.[8] The pars plicata represents the anterior 2 mm, and the pars plana the posterior 4 to 5 mm. If the instrument is too far anterior, it will pass through the pars plicata, increasing the risk of hemorrhage and damage to the lens; if too far posterior, it will perforate the retina, increasing the risk of retinal detachment. If inserted into the region of the pars plana, however, it will penetrate the sclera, connective tissue, pigmented and nonpigmented epithelium, and finally the vitreous—thus decreasing the chance of serious complications.

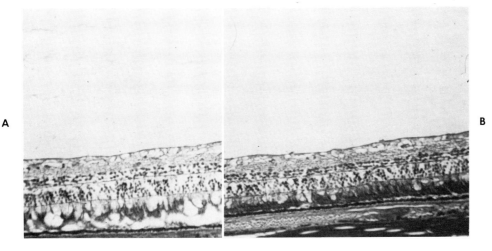

A　　　　　　　　　　　　　　　　　　　　　　　　　　　B

Fig. 1-4. Colloidal iron staining vitreous before and after pretreatment with hyaluronidase. **A,** Colloidal iron stains acid mucopolysaccharides. **B,** No staining occurs after hyaluronidase. (×70; AFIP neg. 57-1284, AFIP acc. no. 778786.) (From Fine, S. S., and Yanoff, M.: Ocular histology, New York, 1972, Harper & Row, Publishers.)

MICROSCOPIC ANATOMY

As previously mentioned, the vitreous is 99% water and is often lost in the preparation of eyes; thus it is difficult to study with light microscopy. By the combined findings of biomicroscopy, electron microscopy, and light microscopy, however, it has been determined to be composed of delicate fibrils—immature collagen. These fibrils are interspersed in a fluid substance which is mostly water but which contains a large amount of hyaluronic acid, as may be demonstrated by the use of special stains for acid mucopolysaccharides (Fig. 1-4).[1,13] The greatest concentration of acid mucopolysaccharides is in the cortical vitreous,[3] because this substance is produced and secreted by the nonpigmented ciliary epithelium in the region of the vitreous base.[2]

Hyalocytes

In the cortical vitreous isolated cells are often found near the surface of the retina (Fig. 1-5). These are called hyalocytes, or vitreous cells, and their exact nature and function have been the topic of considerable research and speculation. Some workers believe these cells may elaborate the hyaluronic acid found within the vitreous.[11] Others think that the hyaluronic acid is elaborated primarily by the nonpigmented ciliary epithelium.[2] According to Fine and Yanoff,[1] more likely the hyalocytes represent histiocytes or glial cells that have migrated from surrounding structures (e.g., the optic nerve head or retinal vessels). They may even be the cells of origin of the preretinal membrane seen in certain pathologic conditions.

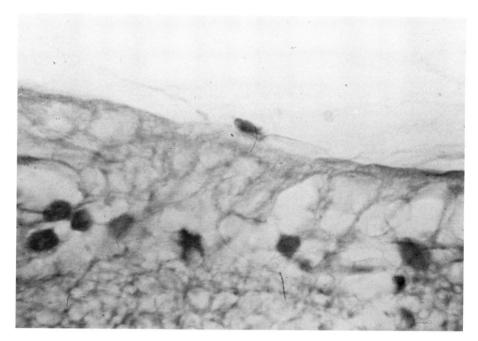

Fig. 1-5. Hyalocyte in cortical vitreous near the surface of the retina (H&E, ×450; AFIP acc. no. 787115).

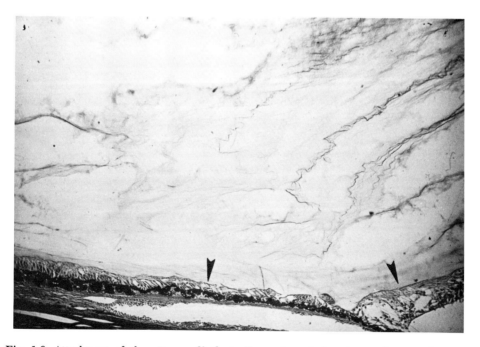

Fig. 1-6. Attachment of the vitreous fibrils in the region of the vitreous base. Left arrow indicates the pars plana epithelium; right arrow the retina (Alcian blue, ×150; AFIP acc. no. 754414).

Attachments

The microscopic attachments of the vitreous gel to adjacent structures may be of considerable importance.[1,4,5] In the region of the vitreous base, the vitreous fibrils appear to emanate from—and may be interwoven with—the basement membrane of the ciliary epithelium (Fig. 1-6), which would account for the firm adherence in this region.[1]

Although the vitreous body is only loosely attached to the internal limiting membrane of the retina, it is often more firmly attached along the course of blood vessels. Porelike defects have been observed in the internal limiting membrane near the blood vessels. Vitreous fibrils may pass through these defects, forming condensations around the blood vessels in the nerve fiber layer[12] and causing the vitreous traction seen to accompany aging. They also may account for the hemorrhages that are sometimes associated with posterior vitreous detachments.

Zonules

The zonules appear microscopically as fine filaments emanating from the basement membrane of the nonpigmented epithelium of the pars plicata. They extend to the equatoral region of the lens and divide so that some fibers attach to the anterior lens capsule and others attach to the posterior lens capsule at the location of the hyaloideocapsular ligament (Fig. 1-7). The zonular fibers that insert more posteriorly into the ora serrata region appear to intermesh with the

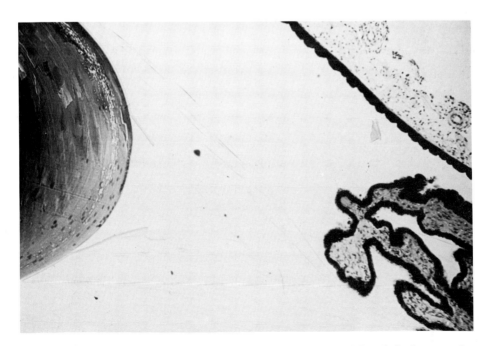

Fig. 1-7. Relationship of zonules to the ciliary processes (on the right) and the lens periphery (on the left) (H&E, ×35; AFIP acc. no. 82691).

basement membrane of the ciliary epithelium, particularly at the apices of the dentate processes.

EMBRYOLOGY

The embryology of the vitreous is described in great detail in textbooks on the subject.[5,10]

Primary vitreous

Briefly the primary vitreous develops during the first month of embryonic life and is derived from *surface ectoderm* in the region of the lens plate, *mesoderm* from the primitive hyaloid system, and *neuroectoderm* from the de-

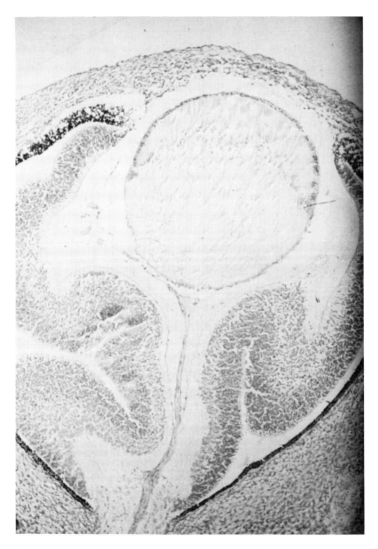

Fig. 1-8. Histologic section of a normal eye from a 9-week embryo. There is vascularized primary vitreous between folds of the developing retina (H&E, × 35; AFIP acc. no. 898149).

veloping retina. It is a highly vascular structure, with the hyaloid vessels spreading out behind the lens to form the posterior vascular tunic of the lens (Fig. 1-8). Its development terminates at about the 13 mm stage when the lens capsule is developing, at which time the surface ectoderm can no longer contribute to its formation.

Secondary vitreous

The secondary vitreous is derived almost entirely from the *developing retina* and is therefore of neuroectodermal origin. It is elaborated by the retina and expands inward to condense the primary vitreous centrally. Eventually the avascular, or adult, vitreous comes to occupy almost all the vitreous cavity. The hyaloid vessels begin to atrophy shortly after the 40 mm stage, and finally the primary vitreous remains only as the condensed walls of the hyaloid canal—surrounded by the adult, or secondary, vitreous.

Tertiary vitreous

The term tertiary vitreous refers to the zonular fibers. These fibers begin as fibrillary outgrowths which emanate from the *basement membrane of the ciliary epithelium* and grow across the marginal bundle of Drault to attach to the equatorial region of the lens.

Regression of the hyaloid system

Shortly after the 40 mm stage, the hyaloid vessels begin to atrophy. This atrophying process commences in the central portion and proceeds anteriorly toward the lens and posteriorly toward the optic disc. Incomplete atrophy of the hyaloid system may account for some of the normal developmental remnants seen in the vitreous. These remnants are usually asymptomatic and may be considered anatomic variations. Mild developmental abnormalities are due to various degrees of persistence of the primary vitreous and include the persistent hyaloid artery, prepapillary vascular loops, Bergmeister's papilla, prepapillary hyaloid cysts, and Mittendorf's dot. Various combinations of entities occur. The more severe variations are discussed in Chapter 2.

DEVELOPMENTAL VARIATIONS
Persistent hyaloid artery

Sometimes the entire hyaloid artery persists as a blood-containing channel or as a fine fibrous cord. It may then appear as a thin linear structure passing from the posterior surface of the lens across the vitreous to the nasal side of the optic disc (Fig. 1-9). When this channel contains blood, it may be the source of vitreous hemorrhage in neonates. In such cases the hemorrhage may be confined to the hyaloid canal, sparing the remainder of the vitreous.

Prepapillary vascular loop

If the hyaloid vessels undergo atrophy centrally but persist posteriorly, they may appear clinically as a prepapillary vascular loop. This loop projects for a

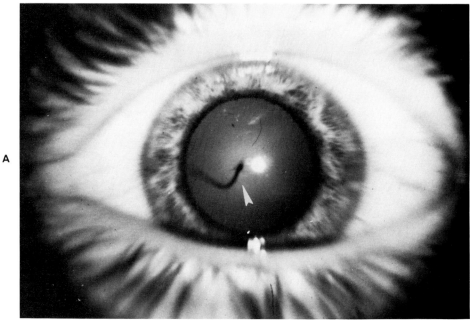

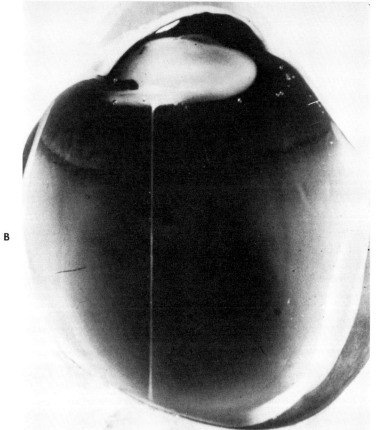

Fig. 1-9. A, Persistent hyaloid artery. Note the attachment to the posterior lens surface (arrow). B, Section of the globe showing the persistent hyaloid artery (AFIP acc. no. 721733). (From Hogan, M. J., and Zimmerman, L. E.: Ophthalmic pathology, Philadelphia, 1962, W. B. Saunders Co.)

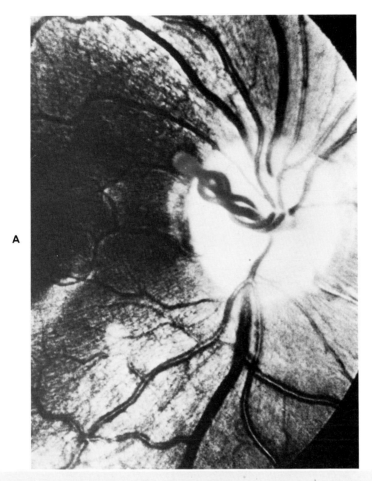

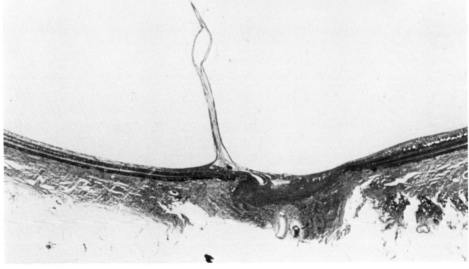

Fig. 1-10. **A,** Prepapillary vascular loop. **B,** Patent vessel projecting anteriorly from the optic disc (H&E, ×30; AFIP acc. no. 118217).

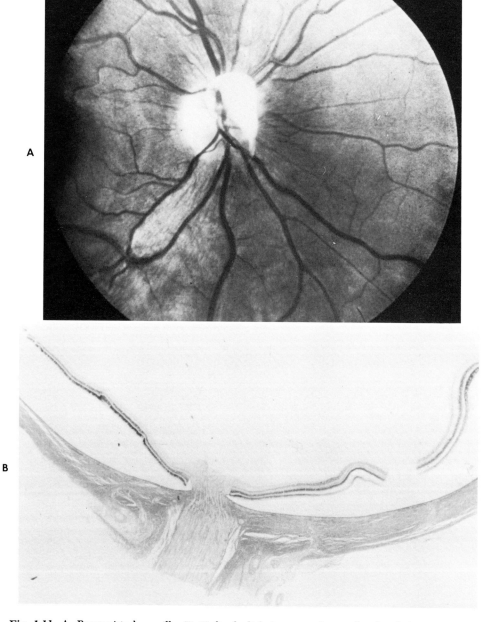

Fig. 1-11. **A,** Bergmeister's papilla. **B,** Tuft of glial tissue on the nasal side of the optic disc (H&E, ×22; AFIP acc. no. 79594).

variable distance into the vitreous and is usually continuous with the retinal vessels at the optic disc (Fig. 1-10).

Bergmeister's papilla

Sometimes the hyaloid vessels disappear, leaving only a tuft of fibroglial tissue at the optic nerve head known as Bergmeister's papilla. Although a number of variations may occur, the papilla usually appears as a yellow-white tuft of connective tissue projecting anteriorly from the nasal side of the optic disc (Fig. 1-11). Occasionally a variant of Bergmeister's papilla is seen with a space between the hyaloid artery and its glial sheath; this space enlarges to form a cyst which appears as a spherical structure over the optic nerve head. Such prepapillary hyaloid cysts may clinically resemble the fossilized astrocytoma seen on the optic disc in patients with tuberous sclerosis.

Mittendorf's dot

Persistence of the hyaloid system at its anterior attachment to the lens may appear as a Mittendorf dot—a small gray opacity just inferonasal to the visual axis on the posterior lens capsule. It is usually asymptomatic and is reported to occur in about 10% of normal patients.[5]

The more severe forms of persistence of the primary vitreous, such as persistent hyperplastic primary vitreous and congenital retinal folds, are pathologic entities that often result in severe visual impairment. These are considered in Chapter 2.

REFERENCES

1. Fine, B. S., and Yanoff, M.: Ocular histology: a text and atlas, New York, 1972, Harper & Row, Publishers.
2. Fine, B. S., and Zimmerman, L. E.: Light and electron microscopic observations on the ciliary epithelium in man and Rhesus monkey, with particular reference to the base of the vitreous body, Invest. Ophthalmol. **2:**105, 1963.
3. Freeman, H. M.: The lens and vitreous, Arch. Ophthalmol. **82:**551, 1969.
4. Hogan, M. J., and Zimmerman, L. E.: Ophthalmic pathology; an atlas and textbook, ed. 2, Philadelphia, 1962, W. B. Saunders Co.
5. Jaffe, N. S.: The vitreous in clinical ophthalmology, St. Louis, 1968, The C. V. Mosby Co.
6. Kasner, D.: Vitrectomy: a new approach to the management of vitreous loss, Highlights Ophthalmol. **11:**304, 1968.
7. McCulloch, C.: The zonule of Zinn: its origin, course, and insertion, and its relationship to neighboring structures, Trans. Am. Ophthalmol. Soc. **52:**525, 1954.
8. Machemer, R.: A new concept for vitreous surgery. II, Surgical technique and complications, Am. J. Ophthalmol. **74:**1022, 1972.
9. Machemer, R., Parel, J. M., and Buettner, H.: A new concept for vitreous surgery. I, Instrumentation, Am. J. Ophthalmol. **73:**1, 1972.
10. Mann, I.: Developmental abnormalities of the eye, Philadelphia, 1957, J. B. Lippincott Co.
11. Szirmai, J. A., and Balazs, E. A.: Studies on the structure of the vitreous body. III, Cells in the cortical layer, Arch. Ophthalmol. **59:**34, 1958.
12. Wolter, J. R.: Pores in the internal limiting membrane of the human retina, Acta Ophthalmol. **42:**971, 1964.
13. Zimmerman, L. E.: Applications of histochemical methods for the demonstration of acid mucopolysaccharides to ophthalmic pathology, Trans. Am. Acad. Ophthalmol. Otolaryngol. **62:**697, 1958.

2

Pathology of the vitreous

JERRY A. SHIELDS

The vitreous is mostly water and is often lost when the eye is routinely sectioned in the laboratory. Consequently it is difficult to study histologically, and many disease processes involving this tissue are not well understood. In the past most knowledge about vitreous pathology has been acquired by studying enucleated eyes or autopsy specimens in which in vivo relationships may be altered. With the recent development of newer surgical instruments for vitrectomy,[11] the vitreous has become accessible to biopsy. Thus further information about the pathologic processes that occur in this portion of the eye may be provided.

The present chapter will consider the pathology of the vitreous in a number of ocular and systemic diseases. Particular emphasis will be placed on conditions that are of concern to the vitreous surgeon.

DEVELOPMENTAL ABNORMALITIES

Most of the developmental abnormalities related to the vitreous are secondary to incomplete atrophy of the fetal hyaloid system, resulting in some degree of persistence of the primary vitreous. These are mainly asymptomatic and of little clinical significance. Two conditions may be of considerable clinical importance, however: persistent hyperplastic primary vitreous (PHPV) and congenital retinal fold. The former is probably related to abnormal vitreous development whereas the pathogenesis of the latter is still a matter of controversy.

Persistent hyperplastic primary vitreous[6,8,17]

Persistent hyperplastic primary vitreous (PHPV) apparently results from an abnormal persistence and proliferation of the posterior tunica vasculosa lentis. The full-blown entity is present at birth and occurs unilaterally in a microphthalmic eye. There is a mild form, characterized by a focal white mass on the posterior lens surface (Fig. 2-1, *A*), and a more severe form, characterized by a larger vascularized retrolental mass into which the ciliary processes may be drawn (Fig. 2-1, *B*). A persistent hyaloid artery is usually present.

14

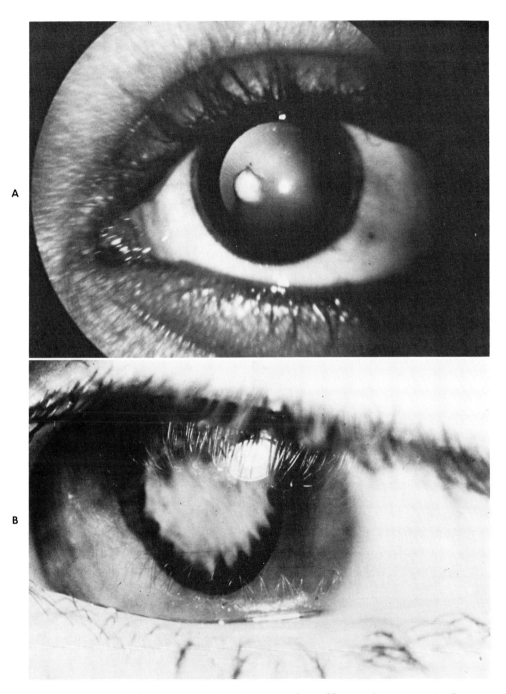

Fig. 2-1. A, Note the focal white retrolental mass in this mild case of PHPV. **B,** In this more severe case, note the large retrolental mass and the elongated ciliary processes. (Courtesy Retina Service, Wills Eye Hospital, Philadelphia.)

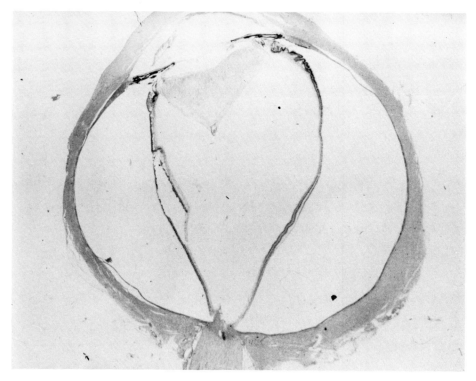

Fig. 2-2. Retrolental fibrovascular mass characteristic of PHPV. Note the partial absence of the lens, the elongated ciliary processes, and the persistent hyaloid vessel (H&E, AFIP acc. no. 786570). (From Hogan, M. J., and Zimmerman, L. E.: Ophthalmic pathology, Philadelphia, 1962, W. B. Saunders Co.)

Pathologically there is a dense retrolental fibrovascular mass. The peripheral portion of the mass may incorporate the ciliary processes as well as the peripheral retina (Fig. 2-2). This is clinically important, because recent reports have emphasized the benefit of surgical excision of the mass.[5] Such surgery should be performed with great care, using the operating microscope to avoid removing portions of the retina.

The lens is usually clear at birth; but often it becomes cataractous when the fibrovascular tissue invades it through dehiscences in the posterior capsule. In later stages of fibrovascular invasion, the lens may spontaneously resorb—leaving only capsular remnants. Recurrent hemorrhages from the fibrovascular mass may then lead to further traction and ultimately cause retinal detachment and glaucoma. Phthisis bulbi has been known to occur in the end stage.

Retinal dysplasia is a common finding in eyes with PHPV. Whether it results from, or predisposes to, PHPV is still uncertain, however. Preretinal glial tissue is a common finding in PHPV and is probably the ectodermal counterpart of the retrolental mesodermal tissue.[14]

PHPV is usually discovered in infancy or childhood. Those cases which have been studied pathologically have been in eyes enucleated with the mistaken

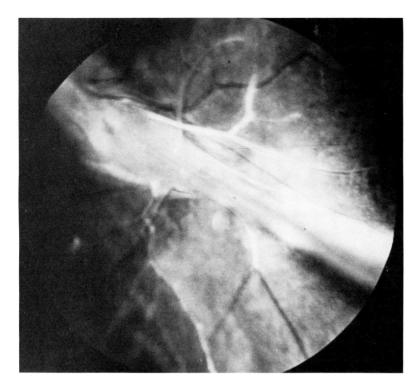

Fig. 2-3. Congenital retinal fold. (Courtesy Retina Service, Wills Eye Hospital, Philadelphia.)

diagnosis of retinoblastoma. More recently cases have been discovered in adulthood, indicating that this abnormality may be mild and may not become significantly symptomatic for a number of years.[19]

Congenital retinal fold

Congenital retinal fold occurs as a band of fibrovascular and glial connective tissue extending from the optic disc across the retina to the ora serrata region (Fig. 2-3). It may occur in any quadrant with equal frequency. Usually called a congenital retinal fold[13] or falciform fold, it is probably identical to posterior hyperplastic primary vitreous.[16]

Pruett and Schepens, in reporting on a series of twelve patients, agreed with Ida Mann that this condition probably results from an abnormal adhesion between the primary vitreous and the retina which prevents the secondary vitreous from compressing these structures centrally.[16] Other authors believe it may represent a variant of retinopathy of prematurity (RLF).

VITREOUS INFLAMMATIONS[6]

Like other tissues of the body, the vitreous may be the site of a number of inflammatory processes. Unlike most other tissues, however, it is avascular and does not respond as do tissues with a blood supply. Certain agents introduced

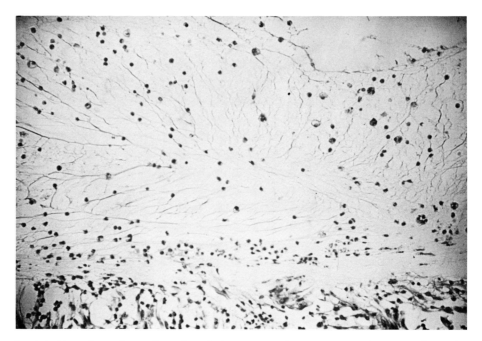

Fig. 2-4. Note the polymorphonuclear leukocytes in the vitreous in this case of purulent endophthalmitis (H&E, ×200; AFIP acc. no. 792134).

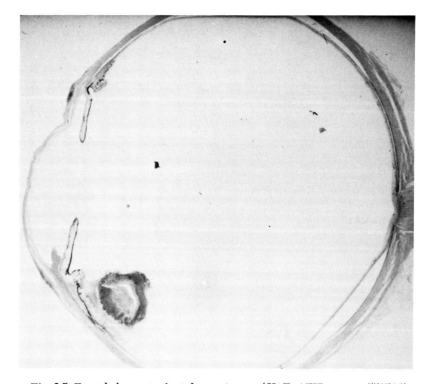

Fig. 2-5. Fungal abscess in the inferior vitreous (H&E, AFIP acc. no. 551747).

into the vitreous may bring about inflammation, varying with the type of agent involved.

Bacterial infections

Pyogenic bacteria (e.g., *Staphylococcus aureus, Pseudomonas aeruginosa*) may produce severe suppurative endophthalmitis, or vitreous abscess, with rapid onset and extensive damage to the intraocular structures. Massive numbers of neutrophils may accumulate within the vitreous cavity (Fig. 2-4).

Mycotic infections

Certain fungal organisms may also provoke a polymorphonuclear response in the vitreous (mycotic endophthalmitis). In contrast to bacterial infections, the mycotic abscess is usually more localized and more slowly progressive. Mycotic abscesses frequently settle to the inferior portion of the vitreous (Fig. 2-5). Fungal stains of vitreous aspirated from such an abscess will reveal the organisms (Fig. 2-6). Because these infections are slowly progressive, they may not become clinically apparent for several days or even weeks after ocular trauma or surgery. Bacterial infections, on the other hand, may be apparent on the first day following surgery.

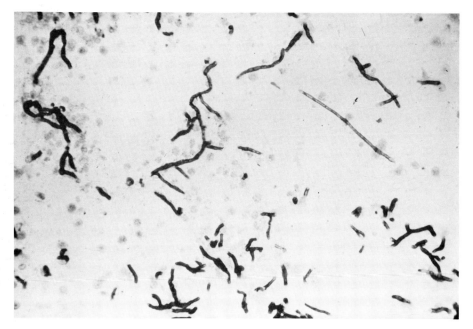

Fig. 2-6. Fungi in a vitreous abscess (Grocott's method, GMS, ×250; AFIP acc. no. 754542).

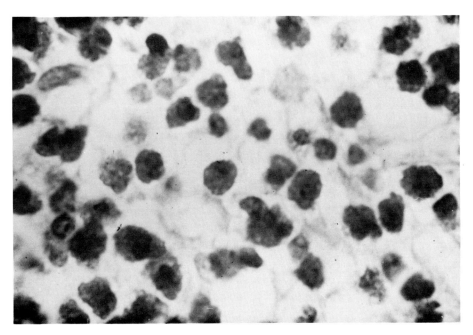

Fig. 2-7. Eosinophils in the vitreous in a case of nematode endophthalmitis due to *Toxocara canis* (H&E, ×600; AFIP acc. no. 298563).

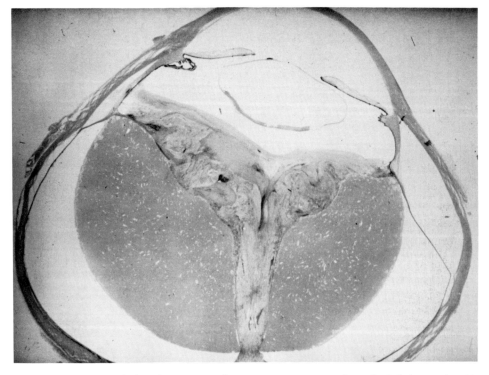

Fig. 2-8. Total retinal detachment secondary to severe nematode endophthalmitis (H&E, AFIP acc. no. 307236).

Parasitic infections

A number of parasites produce an inflammatory reaction in the vitreous. Two of the better-known organisms are the larvae of *Toxocara canis* and *Cysticercus*.

Toxocara may produce either a focal chorioretinal granuloma or a severe reaction with exudation of massive numbers of eosinophils into the vitreous (Fig. 2-7). In the late stages the vitreous may contract and eventually produce a total retinal detachment (Fig. 2-8)—especially in children who have a history of contact with infected dogs.[6]

Cysticercus may form focal white lesions in either the vitreous or the subretinal space.[6] Particularly in tropical areas, a number of other parasitic diseases involve the vitreous.

Miscellaneous inflammations

In addition to the organisms just mentioned, vitreous inflammation can result from other conditions. For example, penetrating ocular injuries and foreign bodies may provoke a chronic inflammatory response with a predominance of lyhphocytes and plasma cells. Certain granulomatous inflammations involving the retina (e.g., toxoplasmosis, idiopathic peripheral uveitis, sarcoidosis) also produce a lymphocytic response in the vitreous by direct extension from areas of retinal involvement.

Sequelae of vitreous inflammation

Mild forms of vitreous inflammation may produce only minor alterations with little residual damage. More severe inflammations, however (e.g., the purulent reactions to bacteria and fungi), may lead to extensive organization with fibrosis and contraction of the vitreous. A cyclitic membrane, incorporating condensed vitreous, new vessels, and proliferated ciliary epithelium, may ensue. On occasion, further contraction of the vitreous has led to total retinal detachment, severe glaucoma, and eventually phthisis bulbi.

VITREOUS HEMORRHAGE[6,8]

Vitreous hemorrhage is a problem commonly encountered by the ophthalmologist. It may occur from the vessels of the retina or ciliary body. True hemorrhage in the vitreous should be differentiated from hemorrhage between the posterior hyaloid face and the retina (subhyaloid, preretinal) and between the nerve fiber layer and internal limiting membrane of the retina (submembranous). Significant hemorrhage into the vitreous framework may lead to organization and vitreous traction whereas subhyaloid or submembranous hemorrhages frequently resolve, leaving very little damage to the vitreous structures.

Etiologies of vitreous hemorrhage

The etiologies of vitreous hemorrhage are too numerous to list here. Such hemorrhage may result from any of a number of congenital, vascular, inflammatory, traumatic, neoplastic, and degenerative conditions.

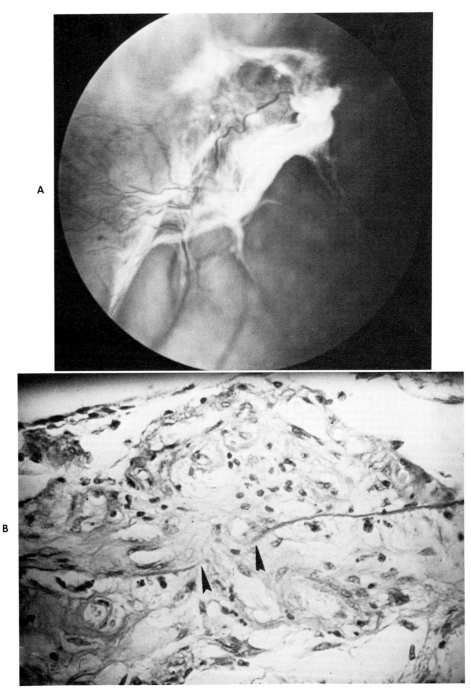

Fig. 2-9. **A,** Preretinal fibrovascular tissue in diabetic retinopathy. **B,** In this case of diabetic retinopathy, the fibrovascular tissue is breaking through the defect in the internal limiting membrane (arrows) (H&E, ×640; AFIP acc. no. 1324019).

Congenital. Several congenital or developmental abnormalities are of particular importance.

A *patent hyaloid artery* may be the source of vitreous hemorrhage in the neonate, especially after blunt trauma, as may occur from the trauma of passing through the birth canal.

In *retinopathy of prematurity* (RLF), vitreous hemorrhage may occur from areas of neovascularization in the peripheral retina—as early or late sequelae of vitreous traction.

Patients with *congenital retinoschisis* may initially present with hemorrhage from the unsupported retinal vessels in the inner layer of the retinoschisis cavity.

As previously mentioned, *persistent hyperplastic primary vitreous* (PHPV) may produce vitreous hemorrhage from either the vascularized retrolental membrane or a persistent hyaloid vessel.

A number of other congenital and developmental conditions also predispose to vitreous hemorrhage.[21]

Acquired. Certain systemic diseases affecting the retinal blood vessels can lead to vitreous hemorrhage.

Perhaps the most important of these is *diabetes mellitus.* In this disorder recurrent hemorrhages occur from areas of preretinal neovascularization. Initially there is retinal neovascularization which may break through the internal limiting membrane of the retina and produce a fibroneovascular growth into the vitreous cavity (Fig. 2-9). As the vitreous gel gradually contracts, these neovascular fronds are pulled anteriorly with the posterior border layer of the vitreous. Most diabetic vitreous hemorrhage therefore actually occurs in a subhyaloid or preretinal location (Fig. 2-10). Recurrent hemorrhage and progressive vitreous contraction may lead to a retinal detachment in the posterior pole characteristic of diabetes (Fig. 2-11).

A similar mechanism occurs in the peripheral retina in *sickle cell disease* and other conditions associated with proliferative retinopathy.

Patients with systemic diseases such as *hypertension,* various *blood dyscrasias, leukemias, polycythemias,* and related conditions may also develop hemorrhage into the vitreous. Occlusion of the central retinal vein or one of its tributaries often later produces preretinal neovascularization and hemorrhage.

Blunt or penetrating ocular injuries may also cause rupture of retinal vessels and vitreous hemorrhage. Traumatic subarachnoid hemorrhage is sometimes associated with peripapillary bleeding into the vitreous.

One of the most important causes of vitreous hemorrhage is a *posterior vitreous detachment*—which may lead to a retinal hole and possible retinal detachment. The retinal break often occurs close to a large retinal vessel (Fig. 2-12). If such a vessel ruptures, vitreous hemorrhage may be the presenting sign of the retinal detachment.

Intraocular tumors do not usually produce significant vitreous hemorrhage. Both retinoblastoma (Fig. 2-13) and malignant melanoma of the choroid occasionally produce bleeding into the vitreous. The hemorrhage may preclude a

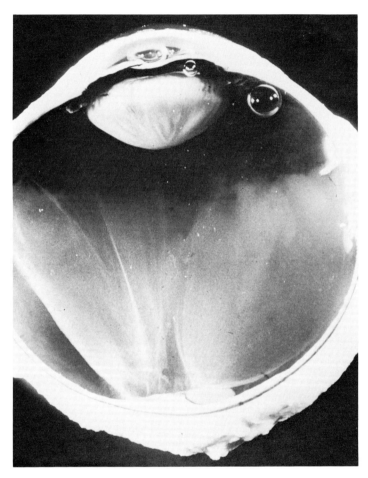

Fig. 2-10. Focal preretinal hemorrhage in a sectioned globe with proliferative diabetic retinopathy (AFIP acc. no. 1089004).

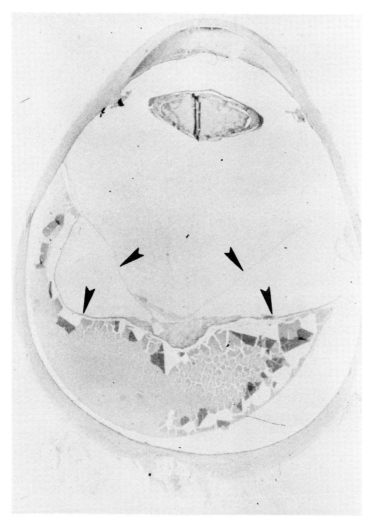

Fig. 2-11. Traction retinal detachment secondary to diabetic retinopathy. Upper arrows indicate the vitreous traction; lower arrows the retina (Wills Eye Hospital Pathology no. 15,982).

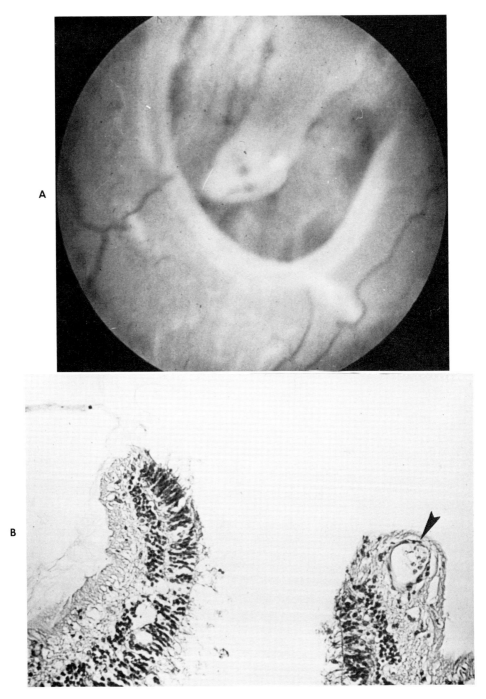

Fig. 2-12. **A,** Horseshoe-shaped retinal tear secondary to vitreous traction. Note the proximity to the retinal vessel. **B,** Retinal break in a similar case. Note the vitreous traction on the operculum (to the left) and the proximity of the retinal vessel (arrow) (Alcian blue, ×200; AFIP acc. no. 859545). (**A** courtesy Retina Service, Wills Eye Hospital, Philadelphia.)

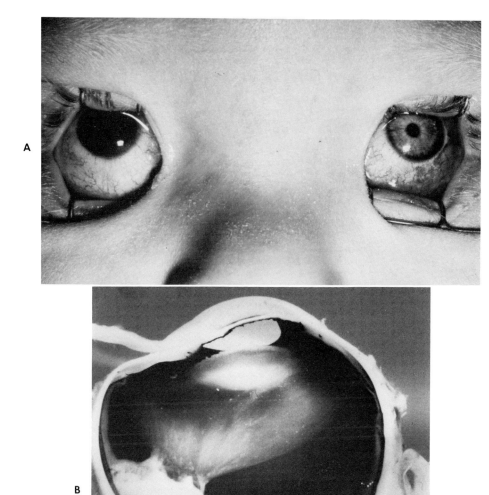

Fig. 2-13. **A,** Dark pupil in the right eye of an infant secondary to vitreous hemorrhage. **B,** In the enucleated right eye there was a retinoblastoma with overlying vitreous detachment and hemorrhage.

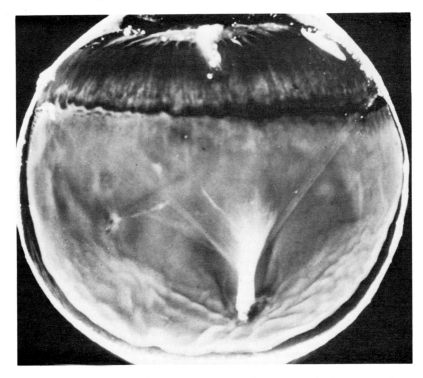

Fig. 2-14. Fibrous traction band in the vitreous of a sectioned globe secondary to organized hemorrhage.

view of the fundus, making the diagnosis more difficult. Retinal angiomas, especially when large, may also cause extensive vitreous hemorrhage.

Sequelae of vitreous hemorrhage

If vitreous hemorrhage is mild, there may be hemolysis of erythrocytes and phagocytosis of blood products by macrophages leading to almost total resolution. If the hemorrhage is more severe, however, the blood may undergo organization—resulting in traction bands (Fig. 2-14) that can eventually produce a retinal hole and detachment. In some cases the breakdown products of blood are deposited in the lens and ciliary epithelia, retina, and dilator and sphincter muscles of the iris, a condition called ocular hemosiderosis[23] which may lead to loss of retinal function and secondary glaucoma.

Another complication of vitreous hemorrhage, rarely diagnosed clinically, is hemolytic glaucoma. In this condition the breakdown products of blood are phagocytosed by macrophages and are carried to the anterior chamber angle, where they produce a mechanical obstruction to aqueous outflow similar to the mechanism of phacolytic glaucoma.[4]

EFFECTS OF TRAUMA ON THE VITREOUS

Pathologic changes in the vitreous can result from blunt or penetrating trauma and from retained intraocular foreign bodies. Ocular injuries may pro-

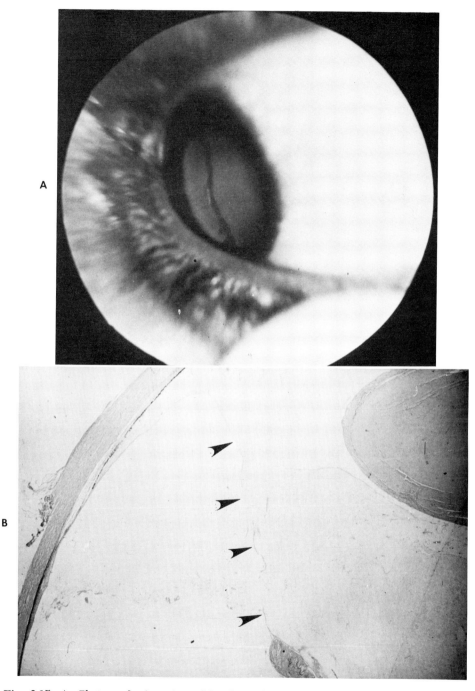

Fig. 2-15. **A,** Photograph through a dilated pupil showing traumatic disinsertion of the vitreous base. **B,** Vitreous base dislocated centrally (arrows) from its usual attachment to the ora serrata region (to the left) (H&E, ×30). (**A** courtesy Retina Service, Wills Eye Hospital, Philadelphia.)

duce hemorrhage, inflammation, and retinal breaks, all of which have been discussed.

A rather characteristic vitreous change after blunt trauma is disinsertion or
avulsion of the vitreous base. At the time of severe ocular contusion (e.g., a blow
to the eye with a fist), there is a sudden equatorial expansion of the ocular
coats. Because the extensibility of the sclera is greater than that of the vitreous
gel, the sclera expands with greater amplitude. As a result the vitreous base
pulls away from its firm attachment and brings with it fragments of the pigmented ciliary epithelium.[22] Clinically the vitreous base can be seen through
the dilated pupil as a linear structure with pigment suspended in the vitreous
cavity (Fig. 2-15, *A*). It oscillates freely with movements of the eye. Histologically the vitreous base is displaced centrally from its usual attachment to the
ora serrata region (Fig. 2-15, *B*). This condition is almost pathognomonic of
ocular trauma and therefore may have both clinical and medicolegal significance.

Penetrating ocular trauma may cause hemorrhage with subsequent fibrosis
and traction bands—often leading to the point of the penetration (Fig. 2-14).

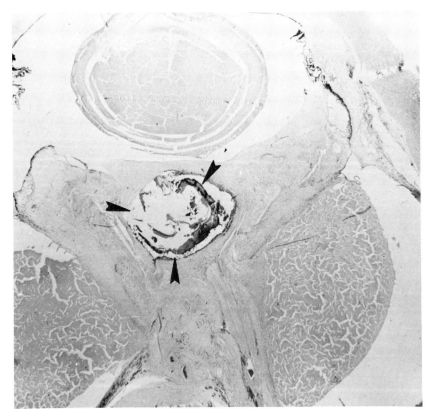

Fig. 2-16. Retained metallic intraocular foreign body in the anterior vitreous (arrows)
causing cataract, cyclitic membrane, and total retinal detachment (H&E, AFIP acc. no.
1337273).

This type of trauma sometimes causes chronic vitreous traction and retinal detachment.

Intraocular foreign bodies may produce vitreous alterations such as hemorrhage, infection, and cataract (Fig. 2-16). Although glass and wooden objects are relatively inert, certain other materials such as copper and iron may produce significant pathologic changes.[17] The widespread distribution of oxidized iron in various parts of the eye leads to a condition called siderosis bulbi, which produces damage to the retina and epithelial structures, secondary glaucoma, and ultimate loss of the eye. Copper foreign bodies may produce changes that vary from a severe inflammatory reaction to the widespread deposition of copper in the eye (chalcosis).[8]

THE VITREOUS IN SYSTEMIC DISEASE

Changes in the vitreous may be associated with a number of systemic diseases. It has already been pointed out that certain vascular diseases, regardless of etiology, produce vitreous hemorrhage. Systemic infections may also spread to involve the vitreous; and certain tumors, such as retinoblastoma and reticulum cell sarcoma, seed their cells into the vitreous. The present section considers primarily the vitreous manifestations of diabetes and amyloidosis, which have received considerable attention in the ophthalmic literature.

Diabetes mellitus

The role of the vitreous in diabetic retinopathy has been alluded to in the section on vitreous hemorrhage. The proliferative form of diabetic retinopathy, however, may lead to profound vitreous alterations—explaining the high incidence of blindness in this disease. Although the underlying stimulus is not clearly understood, the usual sequence of events has been clearly outlined.[2,20] There is at first a proliferation of new vessels along the surface of the retina. These vessels may break through the internal limiting membrane into the vitreous cavity (Fig. 2-9, *B*). Firm adhesions may then develop between the neovascular tissue and the posterior vitreous. Subsequently the vitreous may contract, pulling the new vessels away from the retina. Traction on these new vessels leads to recurrent hemorrhages between the posterior hyaloid face and the retina (Fig. 2-17).

The hemorrhage gradually becomes organized into sheets of fibrous tissue passing from the prepapillary area to the region of the vitreous base. These fibrous sheets may gradually pull the posterior retina anteriorly, leading to a retinal detachment in the posterior pole (Fig. 2-11). Such a tractional detachment with or without a retinal hole is a common occurrence in advanced proliferative retinopathy. Ultimately rubeosis iridis and neovascular glaucoma may ensue.

Primary familial amyloidosis

Amyloidosis is a rare systemic disease of obscure etiology. It is characterized by the deposition of amyloid, a proteinlike substance, throughout the body.[8]

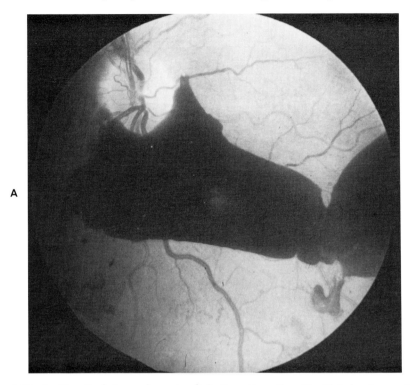

Fig. 2-17. A, Preretinal hemorrhage in diabetic retinopathy. **B,** Globular hemorrhage between the retina and the posterior hyaloid face in a similar case (H&E, ×56; AFIP acc. no. 219451).

The ocular tissues are also susceptible. Falls and co-workers[3] estimated that at least 8% of patients with primary familial amyloidosis have ocular signs and symptoms. Almost every part of the eye may be involved in some way.

The vitreous manifestations of this condition have been the subject of a great deal of ophthalmic interest.[8,9,15] The vitreous gradually becomes filled with white sheetlike opacities that attach to the collagen framework and lead to considerable interference with vision. Although the origin of the amyloid material in the vitreous has been the subject of considerable debate, Wong and McFarlin[25] presented evidence the amyloid may arise from the retinal blood vessels. They examined an 18-year-old woman who had white material extending into the vitreous from a retinal arteriole (Fig. 2-18, *A*). She subsequently died from the renal complications of the disease. Postmortem examination of her eye revealed that the amyloid material in the vitreous was continuous with a pericollagenous focus of amyloid around the retinal vessels (Fig. 2-18, *B*).

With the advent of vitreous biopsy and vitrectomy, the diagnosis and therapy of vitreous amyloidosis have become possible. If the diagnosis is suspected, vitreous biopsy will retrieve the material—which will stain positive with certain fluorescent techniques, Congo red stain, or other methods.[6,8] Total vitrectomy in cases of amyloidosis of the vitreous may offer a good visual prognosis.[9,12]

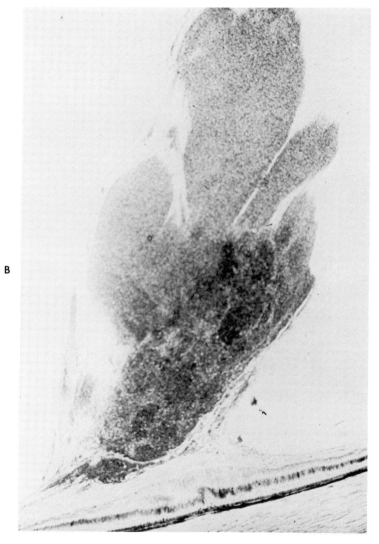

B

Fig. 2-17, cont'd. For legend see opposite page.

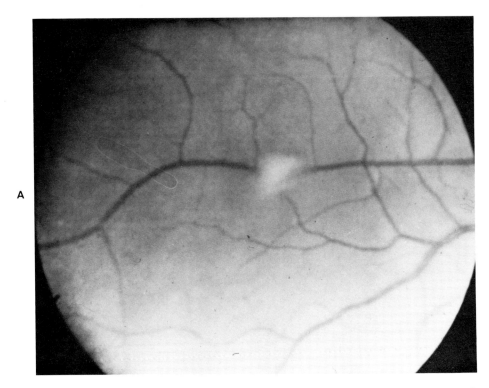

Fig. 2-18. **A,** Primary familial amyloidosis. Note the white material in the vitreous adjacent to the retinal vessel. **B,** Fibrillar amyloid material in the vitreous (above) and around the retinal vessel (below) (Congo red, ×500). (From Wong, V. G., and McFarlin, D. E.: Arch. Ophthalmol. **78:**208, 1967.)

A number of other diseases affect the vitreous secondarily to involvement of the retina. These include granulomatous inflammations such as toxoplasmosis and sarcoidosis, certain fungal and bacterial infections, and tumors.[6]

DEGENERATIVE CONDITIONS OF THE VITREOUS

Degenerative conditions involving the vitreous include changes related to aging, the hereditary hyaloideoretinopathies, and certain miscellaneous conditions of obscure etiology.

Aging changes

The important changes involving the vitreous are liquefaction and posterior vitreous detachment.

With age there is a gradual liquefaction (syneresis) of the vitreous. The process usually begins in the central vitreous as optically clear spaces filled with aqueous-like fluid (Fig. 2-19). These fluid-filled cavities are often lined with condensed vitreous fibrils. Large syneresis cavities in the posterior portion of the vitreous may be confused biomicroscopically with a true posterior vitreous detachment.

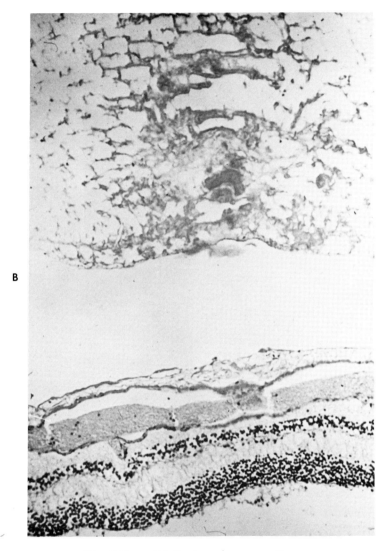

Fig. 2-18, cont'd. For legend see opposite page.

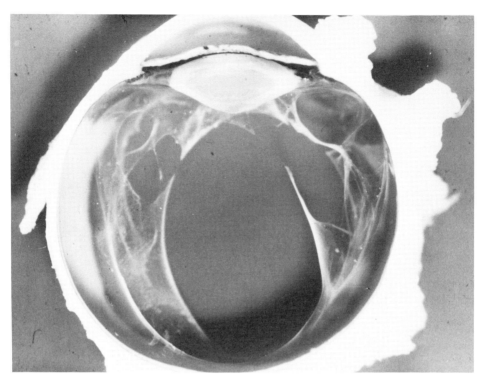

Fig. 2-19. Large syneresis cavities in the central vitreous of a sectioned globe (AFIP acc. no. 137925).

A posterior vitreous detachment is a common finding in older patients, occurring in about 50% of persons over 50 years of age and even more frequently in later years. With increasing age there is a gradual shrinking of the vitreous body so that the posterior hyaloid face separates from the internal limiting membrane of the retina, sometimes with the formation of a condensed cellular membrane on the posterior surface of the detached vitreous (Fig. 2-20). This separation slowly becomes more extensive; and the entire vitreous may peel anteriorly, eventually remaining attached only at the vitreous base.

Jaffe[7,8] points out that there are three main complications of posterior vitreous detachment: vitreous hemorrhage, retinal breaks, and vitreous traction at the posterior pole. As previously mentioned, there may be firm vitreoretinal adhesions at the site of retinal vessels.[24] While the vitreous is separating from the retina, traction at these sites ruptures a retinal vessel. When the vitreous is totally detached, there may be considerable pull on the posterior lip of the vitreous base, particularly in the superior quadrants. Such traction often leads to a retinal tear and retinal detachment.

In some cases of posterior vitreous detachment, residual strands of vitreous may extend to the posterior pole, particularly in the macular region, producing a vitreous traction syndrome. The clinical signs and symptoms are well known

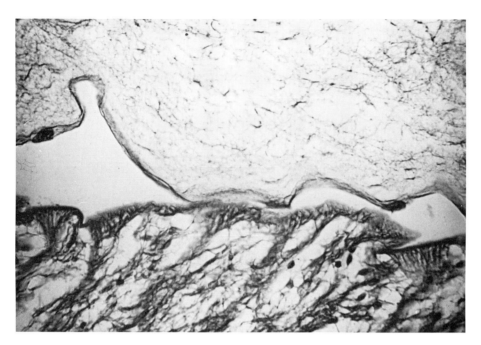

Fig. 2-20. Vitreoretinal interface in early posterior vitreous detachment. Note the cellular membrane on the posterior surface of the detached vitreous (H&E, ×305; AFIP acc. no. 833505). (From Hogan, M. J., and Zimmerman, L. E.: Ophthalmic pathology, Philadelphia, 1962, W. B. Saunders Co.)

to ophthalmologists.[7,8] Pathologically a firm traction band will pull on the macular area (Fig. 2-21) and lead to distortion of the retina.

Hereditary hyaloideoretinopathies

The hereditary hyaloideoretinopathies are rather rare, and good histologic material is not readily available. According to Jaffe[8] the hereditary hyaloideoretinopathies include Wagner's hereditary vitreoretinal degeneration, the hyaloideotapetoretinal degeneration of Goldmann and Favre, and hereditary juvenile retinoschisis. The clinical features of these conditions have been discussed in the literature.[1,8]

Wagner's disease, an autosomal dominant entity, is characterized by progressive liquefaction of the vitreous, peripheral pigmentary degeneration of the retina, and retinoschisis.[1] Goldmann and Favre's disease is simple recessive but may resemble Wagner's disease pathologically.[8] Juvenile retinoschisis is sex-linked recessive and is characterized by marked splitting of the nerve fiber layer with vitreous hemorrhage.[26]

Miscellaneous vitreous degenerations

The miscellaneous category includes myopic vitreoretinal degeneration, asteroid hyalosis, and cholesterosis bulbi.

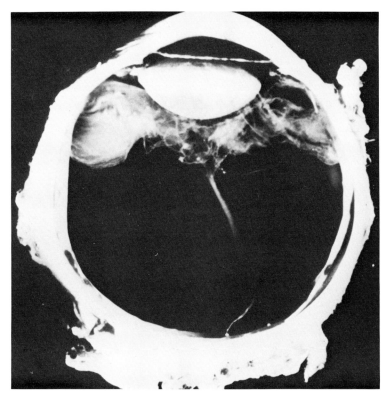

Fig. 2-21. Posterior vitreous detachment with a residual strand of vitreous extending posteriorly to the macula.

In myopia the clinical and histologic features of the vitreous changes are probably no different from those that occur with aging, but they occur at an earlier age than in the nonmyopic population.

Asteroid hyalosis (Benson's disease) is a striking clinical condition characterized by brilliant yellow intravitreal opacities. With the slit lamp microscope they may resemble a galaxy of stars within the vitreous, explaining their name (Fig. 2-22, *A*). In the freshly sectioned eye they appear as distinct particles attached to the vitreous framework (Fig. 2-22, *B*).

Rodman and co-workers[18] studied the histology of asteriod hyalosis in a series of enucleated autopsy eyes. They concluded that these bodies are composed of calcium-containing lipid, as suggested by previous workers.

Microscopically asteroid hyalosis stains lightly with hematoxylin-eosin (Fig. 2-22, *C*) and is typically birefringent under polarized light. The hyalosis also stains positive for lipid and calcium. The exact pathogenesis of these bodies, however, is still poorly understood. Although they were once thought to be closely related to diabetes mellitus, recent studies have suggested that there is no relationship between asteroid hyalosis and diabetes or abnormal plasma lipid levels.[10]

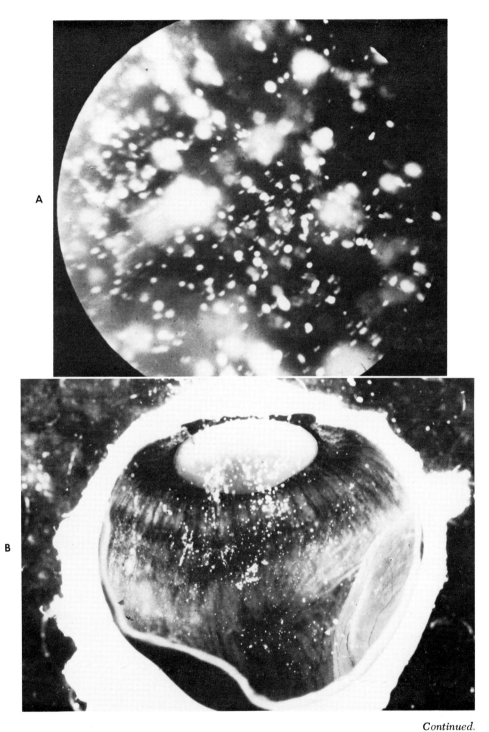

Continued.

Fig. 2-22. **A**, Asteroid hyalosis. Note the refractile bodies in the vitreous. **B**, Section of the eye with asteroid hyalosis showing the numerous asteroid bodies attached to the vitreous fibrils. The eye was enucleated for unrelated malignant melanoma of the choroid.

C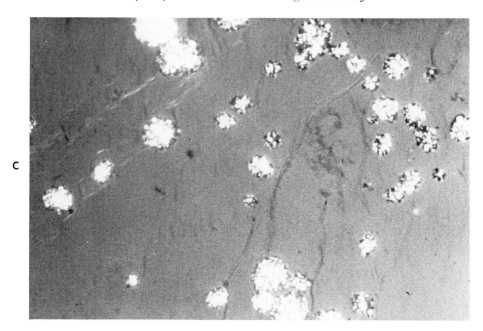

Fig. 2-22, cont'd. C, Asteroid bodies in vitreous (H&E, ×100).

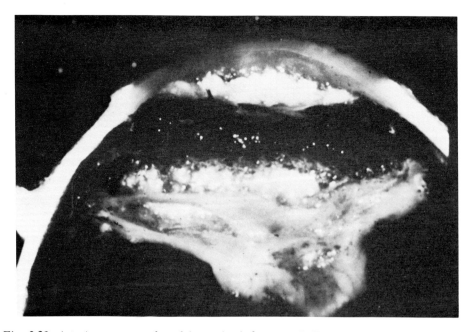

Fig. 2-23. Anterior segment of a globe with cholesterosis bulbi. Note the white glistening bodies in the anterior vitreous and the anterior chamber. There is marked disorganization of the anterior chamber due to previous trauma.

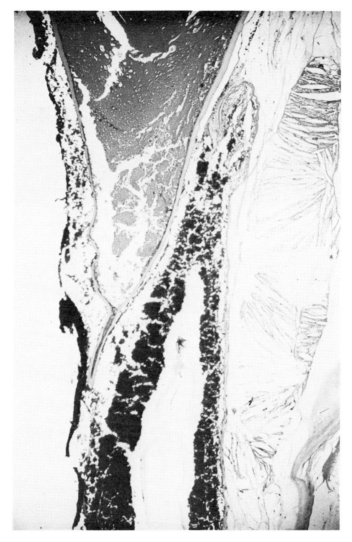

Fig. 2-24. Traumatic cataract and hemorrhage (to the left) and cholesterol clefts in the anterior vitreous (to the right) in an eye with cholesterosis bulbi (H&E, ×100; AFIP acc. no. 929200).

A condition sometimes confused with asteroid hyalosis is cholesterosis bulbi, previously referred to as synchysis scintillans. In this condition clinically there are white particles within the vitreous, and frequently in the anterior chamber as well (Fig. 2-23). In contrast to asteroid hyalosis, the particles are not attached to the vitreous framework but rather appear to float freely in a liquefied vitreous. Cholesterosis bulbi is reported to occur in eyes with a history of trauma, hemorrhage, or inflammation, whereas asteroid hyalosis usually occurs in otherwise normal eyes.[6,8] Histologically, as the name implies, the white particles in cholesterosis bulbi consist of cholesterol. They are often dissolved in formalin fixation, leaving only the characteristic slitlike spaces (Fig. 2-24).

REFERENCES

1. Alexander, R. L., and Shea, M.: Wagner's disease, Arch. Ophthalmol. **74**:310, 1965.
2. Davis, M. D.: Vitreous contraction in proliferative diabetic retinopathy, Arch. Ophthalmol. **74**:741, 1965.
3. Falls, H. F., Jackson, J., Carey, J. H., Rukavina, J. G., and Block, W. D.: Ocular manifestations of hereditary primary systemic amyloidosis, Arch. Ophthalmol. **54**:660, 1955.
4. Fenton, R. H., and Zimmerman, L. E.: Hemolytic glaucoma, Arch. Ophthalmol. **70**:148, 1963.
5. Gass, J. D. M.: Surgical excision of persistent hyperplastic primary vitreous, Arch. Ophthalmol. **83**:163, 1970.
6. Hogan, M. J., and Zimmerman, L. E.: Ophthalmic pathology; an atlas and textbook, ed. 2, Philadelphia, 1962, W. B. Saunders Co.
7. Jaffe, N. S.: Complications of acute posterior vitreous detachment, Arch. Ophthalmol. **79**:568, 1968.
8. Jaffe, N. S.: The vitreous in clinical ophthalmology, St. Louis, 1969, The C. V. Mosby Co.
9. Kasner, D., Miller, G. R., Taylor, W. H., Sever, R. J., and Norton, E. W. D.: Surgical treatment of amyloidosis of the vitreous, Trans. Am. Acad. Ophthalmol. Otolaryngol. **72**:410, 1968.
10. Luxenberg, M., and Sime, D.: Relationship of asteroid hyalosis to diabetes mellitus and plasma lipid levels, Am. J. Ophthalmol. **67**:406, 1969.
11. Machemer, R., Parel, J. M., and Buettner, H.: A new concept for vitreous surgery. I, Instrumentation, Am. J. Ophthalmol. **73**:1, 1972.
12. Machemer, R., Parel, J. M., and Buettner, H.: A new concept for vitreous surgery. III, Indications and results, Am. J. Ophthalmol. **74**:1, 1972.
13. Mann, I.: Congenital retinal folds, Br. J. Ophthalmol. **19**:641, 1935.
14. Manschot, W. A.: Persistent hyperplastic primary vitreous, Arch. Ophthalmol. **59**:188, 1958.
15. Paton, D., and Duke, J. R.: Primary familial amyloidosis, Am. J. Ophthalmol. **61**:736, 1966.
16. Pruett, R. C., and Schepens, C. L.: Posterior hyperplastic primary vitreous, Am. J. Ophthalmol. **69**:535, 1970.
17. Reese, A. B.: Tumors of the eye, ed. 2, New York, 1963, Harper & Row, Publishers.
18. Rodman, H. I., Johnson, F. B., and Zimmerman, L. E.: New histological and histochemical observations concerning asteroid hyalitis, Arch. Ophthalmol. **66**:552, 1969.
19. Spaulding, A. G.: Persistent hyperplastic primary vitreous humor. A finding in a 71-year-old man, Survey Ophthalmol. **12**:448, 1968.
20. Tasman, W. S.: Retinal detachment secondary to proliferative diabetic retinopathy, Arch. Ophthalmol. **87**:286, 1972.
21. Tasman, W. S., editor: Retinal diseases in children, New York, 1971, Harper & Row, Publishers.
22. Weidenthal, D. T., and Schepens, C. L.: Peripheral fundus changes associated with ocular contusion, Am. J. Ophthalmol. **62**:465, 1966.
23. Winter, F. C.: Ocular hemosiderosis, Trans. Am. Acad. Ophthalmol. Otolaryngol. **71**:813, 1967.
24. Wolter, J. R.: Pores in the internal limiting membrane of the human retina, Acta Ophthalmol. **42**:971, 1964.
25. Wong, V. G., and McFarlin, D. E.: Primary familial amyloidosis, Arch. Ophthalmol. **78**:208, 1967.
26. Yanoff, M., Rahn, E. K., and Zimmerman, L. E.: Histopathology of juvenile retinoschisis, Arch. Ophthalmol. **79**:49, 1968.

3

Operative loss of vitreous

NORMAN S. JAFFE

Aside from expulsive hemorrhage, loss of vitreous is the most serious ocular complication that occurs during cataract surgery. Its importance is underscored by the fact that it is largely preventable.

The past twenty-five years have been marked by significant progress in reducing the incidence of operative loss of vitreous. Surgeons whose experience spans this period can bear adequate testimony to the validity of the statement. It is difficult to appreciate from the literature the progress that has been made. Reports abound on the incidence of vitreous loss during cataract surgery and the measures recommended to prevent such occurrence. When one reads these surveys, dating back to the middle of the 19th century and arising from centers all over the world, a sense of frustration arises if one attempts to draw meaningful conclusions. The variables are so numerous that these surveys educate us very little.

Nevertheless, the results of cataract surgery have markedly improved and the incidence of operative loss of vitreous has sharply declined. It would be of interest to investigate the reasons for the lessened rate of vitreous loss; however, some of the variables that influence all large statistical surveys of complications of cataract surgery should first be discussed.

The first variable concerns the surgeon—whose surgical ability, era of education, locale, and reputation for accurate and objective reporting of his results must all be considered.

The second variable involves the predominant type of patient in the survey. Private patients generally are easier to follow, obey instructions better, and report complicating symptoms more readily than do other patients. In countries where poverty and malnutrition predominate, patients are more likely to lower the incidence of surgical success.

Taken in part from Jaffe, N. S.: Cataract surgery and its complications, St. Louis, 1972, The C. V. Mosby Co.

43

Another variable is the institution in which the surgery is performed. Modern facilities supply more and better operating room personnel, equipment, and postoperative care than do less well-equipped hospitals. In addition, medical records are likely to be kept in an orderly manner. It would be difficult to compare the nursing care in any modern first-rate hospital with that in some of the antiquated facilities in poverty-stricken areas. Considerations such as these too numerous to list tend to influence the statistics in most surveys.

An additional variable in comparing the results of older authors with those of modern series is that the former usually included planned extracapsular extractions. Some series relate the incidence of operative loss of vitreous in all types of lens extractions, including those in eyes with dislocated lenses.

The experience of Vail[43] and Barraquer[3] probably reflect most accurately the progress made in recent years. Vail reported a 12.7% incidence of loss of vitreous in 1,601 cataract extractions from 1925 to 1942. In a subsequent series of 1,292 such operations performed by Shoch and Vail between 1946 and 1961, the rate of operative loss of vitreous fell to 3.7%—an almost 350% decline. Barraquer's rate of vitreous loss fell from 7.3% in 1945 to less than 1% at present.

It is probably fair to state that an incidence of vitreous loss of about 3% should be attained because of the major improvements that have occurred in surgical training, techniques, instrumentation, and facilities. This figure is likely to drop even further as more surgeons become aware of and utilize these improvements.

The importance of preventing operative loss of vitreous has been known for a long time, as evidenced by the following 200-year-old statement by A. G. Richter,[36] of Germany:

> I confess that I have seen this accident [loss of vitreous] happen but very seldom during the operation, and when it does so, there is always some particular cause for it. Either the assistant who supports the eye-lids presses unguardedly on the eye itself or the operator performs his part so awkwardly that the eye is violently irritated or injured, or he makes use of a bad method of operating, or his instruments are ill adapted for the intended purposes, or he persists in his endeavors to force out the lens although he has made the incision in the cornea too small, or he presses hard on the eye without having previously punctured the capsule.
>
> These are circumstances which the operator must avoid if he means to prevent the discharge of the vitreous humor.

In commenting on Richter's observation, Vail[43] noted that this "remarkable statement of two centuries ago leaves us little to add to the subject of prevention. It is particularly to be noted that Richter rightly puts the blame upon the operator and not the patient."

Ironically the serious import of operative loss of vitreous has been emphasized only during the past twenty-five years, during which time the greatest strides toward its prevention have been made. Whereas earlier writers[41,45] had implied that a small or moderate loss of vitreous was of little or no consequence, Vail[43] —in the Gifford lecture of 1964—observed that deleterious results are common and loss of vitreous can indeed have very grave consequences. It also matters little whether a small or a moderate amount of vitreous has been lost.

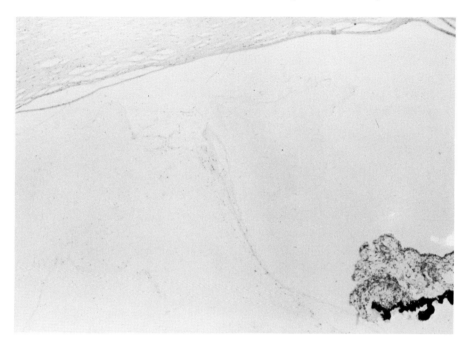

Fig. 3-1. Direct contact of vitreous with the back of the cornea after cataract extraction. (From Jaffe, N. S.: Cataract surgery and its complications, St. Louis, 1972, The C. V. Mosby Co.)

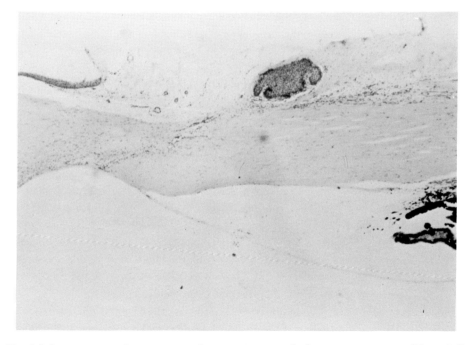

Fig. 3-2. Incarceration of vitreous into the operative wound after cataract surgery. (From Jaffe, N. S.: Cataract surgery and its complications, St. Louis, 1972, The C. V. Mosby Co.)

CONSEQUENCES OF OPERATIVE LOSS OF VITREOUS

The complications that result from operative loss of vitreous are not at all related to the loss of vitreous bulk itself but to the morphologic changes in the vitreous body that occur when the anterior hyaloid membrane is ruptured. These complications are thus related to the following mechanisms:

1. Direct contact of the vitreous with other structures (e.g., the cornea) (Fig. 3-1)
2. Incarceration of vitreous into the operative wound (Fig. 3-2)
3. Fibroplasia of the residual vitreous
4. Inflammation

Most consequences of vitreous loss may be explained by one of the foregoing mechanisms. A list of the important complications would include the following.

Excessive astigmatism. Excessive astigmatism is undoubtedly related to defects of wound healing when vitreous adheres to the operative site.

Bullous keratopathy. The normal cornea may tolerate apposition of vitreous fibrils to its posterior surface; but if the endothelial cell population is sparse because of dystrophy or surgical trauma, a persistent corneal edema with bullous formation may result.

Epithelial invasion of the anterior chamber. As a result of incarceration or prolapse of vitreous into or through the surgical wound, surface epithelium may be encouraged to enter the anterior chamber. If contact with uveal tissue and a plasmoid aqueous humor occurs, an epithelial cyst or a downgrowth of epithelium as a sheet over the cornea and iris may result.

Fibrous ingrowth. An ingrowth of stromal elements may result from a similar mechanism or from fibrous metaplasia of endothelial cells due to vitreous adherence to the wound.

Wound infection and endophthalmitis. The presence of vitreous fibrils between the lips of the wound delays healing and may provide a portal into the eye for pathogenic organisms. This is more likely if the conjunctival coverage of the wound is defective, as may occur with a retracted fornix-based flap.

Iris prolapse. If vitreous fibrils between the lips of the wound delay healing, external pressure on the globe (squeezing or rubbing) may favor an iris prolapse.

Updrawn or misshapen pupil. As a result of fibroplasia, the pupil may be severely distorted and result in a hammock pupil—which may interfere with contact lens fitting. The pupil in some cases may actually be completely covered by the upper eyelid.

Fibroplastic traction bands. Fibroplastic traction bands that connect the posterior surface of the operative wound to other structures such as the retina and ciliary body may cause a retinal detachment or an intense uveitis.

Secondary glaucoma. Glaucoma may be the result of anterior synechiae or chronic irritation and is due to fibroplasia of the damaged vitreous.

Cystoid macular edema and papilledema. The incidence of postoperative cystoid macular edema and papilledema rises sharply when vitreous loss occurs;

and they persist for longer periods of time than when the anterior face of the vitreous is intact. The final result may be a permanent degeneration of the macula with subnormal visual acuity.

Vitreous opacities. In addition to whitish fiberlike membranes in the anterior chamber, vitreous opacities are often found more posteriorly. They may also be associated with hemorrhage or uveitis.

Vitreous hemorrhage. Bleeding into the vitreous is a common accompaniment of operative loss of vitreous. Whether this is caused by separation of angiovitreal adhesions or by loss of vascular support is not known.

Expulsive hemorrhage. The rare but destructive complication of expulsive hemorrhage may occur more frequently when vitreous is lost at the time of surgery.

Fibroplastic condensation of the residual formed vitreous. Fibroplastic condensation may obstruct vision or may cause aphakic pupillary block. The new membrane is occasionally very thick and vascularized. It may prevent free passage of water and electrolytes through its anterior surface.

Retinal detachment. The incidence of retinal detachment after cataract extraction increases greatly in those eyes that suffer operative loss of vitreous.

Chronic ocular irritability. An eye that has lost vitreous at the time of surgery often remains inflamed, tears frequently, and is intensely photophobic. Even a drop of topical anesthetic solution placed in such an eye may cause marked redness.

The large number of described sequelae resulting from a single operative complication should be adequate reason for all ophthalmologists to direct their efforts to the prevention of operative loss of vitreous.

FOLLOW-UP OF EYES WITH OPERATIVE LOSS OF VITREOUS

Few reports exist in the ophthalmic literature on the long-term follow-up of patients who have suffered operative loss of vitreous. Three carefully documented reports[16,43,44] (Vail and Dunphy) show a striking agreement in the average final visual acuity, 20/56. Most of the complications related to vitreous loss occur during the first year after cataract surgery. Vail showed that 6% of these eyes were totally lost within the first few months after surgery and about 23% of the surviving eyes had no useful vision at the end of two years. Furthermore, only 20% of eyes that survived after three years had a vision of 20/70 or better.

In a long-term follow-up of these patients, he concluded that if the eye remained quiet for two or three years after surgery the chance for maintenance of useful vision for the rest of the patient's life was very good—as good, perhaps, as if no vitreous had been lost—subject, of course, to the usual attrition of age.

These series are now obsolete because of significant improvements in the management of operative loss of vitreous. Long-term follow-ups of the newer methods are becoming available.

RECOGNITION OF THE DANGEROUS EYE
Before surgery

A history of operative loss of vitreous in the opposite eye or, in the absence of a history, clinical signs of loss of vitreous should alert the surgeon to take extra precautions when operating on the second eye. Sometimes, despite every prophylactic measure, the same complication results. The chance of vitreous loss in the second eye is probably much greater if operative loss of vitreous befell the first eye. Such loss may be related to an ocular structural deformity present in both eyes (e.g., lack of scleral rigidity, which permits the walls of the globe to collapse when the eye is decompressed), an inherent weakness in the anterior hyaloid membrane, or some other unknown cause.

The physical and mental condition of the patient may be such that accidental loss of vitreous can be anticipated, yet surgery should not be postponed if the condition is chronic. One might include such conditions as marked obesity, diabetes of long standing, advanced arteriosclerosis with vascular hypertension, a history of infection, a bleeding tendency, malnutrition, bronchial asthma, emphysema, chronic bronchitis, chronic cough, mental agitation, and psychosis. There is no real evidence, however, that some of these conditions are related to operative loss of vitreous.

The findings during the examination of the patient that may alert the surgeon to the possibility of vitreous loss include proptosis (especially when associated with increased orbital resistance), glaucoma, evidence of previous intraocular surgery, high myopia, subluxated or dislocated lens, eyelid abnormalities (e.g., shortening of the palpebral fissure), conjunctival abnormalities such as essential shrinkage, and a short thick neck. Theoretically venous pressure is increased in such patients when they are placed in a prone position. This may cause external pressure on the globe.

Measures to prevent loss of vitreous

Readjustment of preoperative medication and choice of anesthesia. A combination of drugs to produce sedation, analgesia, tranquility, and antiemesis should be selected according to the needs of the patient. A choice of anesthesia (local, general, or a combination of both) should be selected not only to suit the patient but also to suit the temperament of the surgeon under the condition encountered.

Surgery on the soft eye. Soft-eye surgery is in my opinion the single most important factor developed during the past twenty-five years to reduce the incidence of vitreous loss. The soft eye may be achieved by three methods: digital ocular compression, hyperosmotic agents, and posterior sclerotomy.

DIGITAL OCULAR COMPRESSION. The principal method of achieving the soft eye is the application for 5 or more minutes of digital pressure (relaxed intermittently to prevent vascular occlusion) after a retrobulbar injection of anesthetic solution (Fig. 3-3).

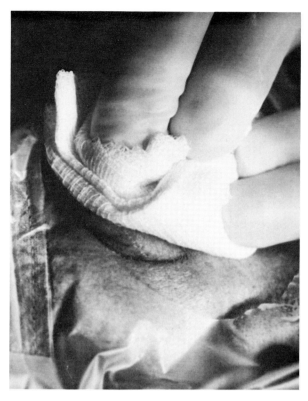

Fig. 3-3. Digital pressure. (From Jaffe, N. S.: Cataract surgery and its complications, St. Louis, 1972, The C. V. Mosby Co.)

Although the ancient Greeks used massage of the eye therapeutically,[13] whether they realized that the eye softened from the massage is not known. We are certain that the effects of digital ocular compression in lowering intraocular pressure date back at least to the nineteenth century.[15,34]

In more recent times digital ocular compression has been used for other reasons. Atkinson[2] recommended it to ensure a more thorough diffusion of anesthetic solution within the muscular cone after a retrobulbar injection. It has been used as a tamponade against any possible bleeding after the retrobulbar injection. Although the originator of the idea was unknown to me, I used it for this purpose before learning of its hypotensive advantages. Chandler is generally credited with employing digital ocular compression after the retrobulbar injection to lower the IOP during cataract surgery.

Kirsch and Steinman[26] were primary instigators in popularizing the technique. Kirsch became interested in it after observing its use by Chandler of Boston. They lauded its benefits as a result of an excellent study that clearly demonstrated its pressure-lowering qualities, both by tonometric measurement and by clinical observation during cataract extraction. They reported a profound decrease in intraocular pressure to an average of 2.3 mm Schiøtz in 100 cases. The average duration of pressure below 10 mm was 14.3 minutes. This short span of hypotension must be kept in mind so the incision will be made during the low-pressure interval.

I have been influenced greatly by Kirsch and Steinman in applying this method during cataract surgery. It has resulted in decreased tonometric readings accompanied by the clinical signs of profound hypotony—lessened tendency for wound gape or spontaneous iris prolapse after the cataract incision, central corneal collapse, marked concavity of the anterior face of the vitreous after the lens is extracted, spontaneous filling of the anterior chamber with air as the lens is delivered.

The mechanism for the hypotony induced by digital massage is not completely clear, which merely means the "mechanism" has received less attention than that accorded hyperosmotic agents; but the evidence points to the escape of fluid from the vitreous as the probable cause.

Hildreth[22] studied the effects of digital ocular compression and considered the induced hypotony to be caused mainly by loss of fluid from the vitreous, plus expression of aqueous. Support for this thesis is furnished by the difficulties encountered in softening the eyes of children by digital massage. The vitreous in such eyes may have undergone little or no liquefaction as in the senile eye.

Further evidence was supplied by Quinn and Porter,[35] who in 1963 used tritiated water in experiments on dogs and observed that less water remained in the vitreous of the massaged globes.

Using a technique of weighing the vitreous after digital compression, Robbins and co-workers[37] found a reduction in vitreous weight and volume in rabbits sufficient to explain the hypotony induced.

In a more recent report François and his co-workers[18] reported that digital massage caused a decrease in IOP, especially in adults and elderly patients. They noted that there was no change in the depth of the anterior chamber—which argues in favor of the arrival of fluid from the vitreous as fast as aqueous is expelled from the anterior chamber. They also noted a decreased concentration of glucose and phosphate in the aqueous, and they attributed this observation to the dilution of these agents by water from the vitreous. Using experimental methods, they observed that the sclera, uvea, retina, lens, and anterior chamber weighed more after digital massage but the vitreous weighed less. They concluded that, although the quantity of water chemically linked to the macromolecular structures of the vitreous varies little, it is the free or non-linked water which is eliminated. They pointed to Schlemm's canal and the vitreous base as exit sites. Thus they also attributed the hypotensive effect of digital massage to the elimination of fluid from the eye.

From the practical point of view, we should not lose sight of what we are trying to accomplish with digital massage. Are we trying to lower the intraocular pressure or reduce the vitreous volume? The argument has been made that digital pressure is of little benefit since the intraocular pressure falls to 0 as soon as the globe is opened. Thus it is not the intraocular pressure but the volume of vitreous which is important.

Would we consider the performance of a cataract extraction safe on an eye with an intraocular pressure of 80 mm Hg since the pressure falls to atmospheric as soon as the incision is made? If not, why not? Perform the following experiment on two eye bank eyes: Using a 30-gauge needle, inject 0.5 ml of water into the vitreous of one eye through the posterior portion of the sclera. This will make the eye extremely hard. Make an incision into the anterior chamber of both globes. Note the forward propulsion of intraocular contents in the hard eye compared to the soft eye. In clinical practice I have observed that eyes with hypotony due to previously performed fistulizing operations may show a tendency to vitreous bulge during cataract surgery if not subjected to digital pressure after the retrobulbar injection. We should also be able to see that a greater force is required against the globe from without to create a vitreous bulge if vitreous volume is previously decreased.

Although the foregoing arguments appear to minimize the factor of lowering IOP, the intraocular pressure is nonetheless an important monitor of what is happening within the globe during digital massage. Indeed, I use digital ocular compression in every cataract extraction. Instead of exerting the pressure for a fixed period of time and then measuring IOP, however, I use a sterile autoclavable Schiøtz tonometer to make frequent measurements during the massage period. I have occasionally observed that the intraocular pressure actually rises during the first minute. Whether this is caused by displacing some of the aqueous into the vitreous I do not know. In most eyes the pressure during the second minute falls precipitously. I have found that eyes whose intraocular pressures can be massaged to a scale reading of 12 or greater with a 5.5-gram weight in 2 minutes or less usually contain a markedly dehydrated vitreous. If at least 5 minutes are required to achieve hypotony, a dangerous situation exists. These eyes may not show the clinical evidence of hypotony after the globe is opened. In these the added precaution of a posterior sclerotomy is sometimes taken.

To this point no mention has been made of the effect of digital massage on orbital volume. The reduction of orbital volume is probably equally as important as the reduction of vitreous volume. It should be apparent that if there is less mass exerting external pressure against the open globe there will be less likelihood of operative loss of vitreous. To quantitate the reduction of orbital volume is difficult, but there is adequate clinical evidence that such reduction occurs. Note the increasing enophthalmos as digital pressure continues—a comforting as well as practical sign of the reduction of orbital volume.

An interesting observation was made by Curtin,[14] who recommended an alternative to digital ocular compression. He used a Schiøtz tonometer with a 10-gram load and placed it on the cornea to obtain a scale reading of 0 (81.7 mm Hg). In 2 minutes the pressures of 70% of the eyes fell to 0, and 50% of these showed off-the-scale readings in 4 minutes. He attributed this hypotensive effect to the absence of compression of the episcleral veins that occurs to some extent with digital massage. The Schiøtz tonometer technique also avoids eyelid gland massage. Nevertheless only half the eyes undergoing cataract extraction showed a concave anterior vitreous face immediately after lens extraction. All patients were operated on under general anesthesia, and no retrobulbar injections were performed. My impression is that the Schiøtz tonometer technique is an effective method of reducing intraocular pressure but is less efficient in reducing orbital volume.

Other benefits of digital ocular compression, as mentioned earlier, include a more thorough diffusion of the anesthetic agent within the muscular cone and probably some hemostasis after the retrobulbar injection. The benefits can be summarized as follows:

1. Decrease of vitreous volume
2. Decrease of orbital volume
3. Better akinesia and anesthesia
4. Hemostasis within the orbit

HYPEROSMOTIC AGENTS. In recent years the efficacy of hyperosmotic agents in reducing intraocular pressure has been applied to reducing some of the hazards of intraocular surgery. That these agents could be employed effectively to lower intraocular pressure has been known for some time. Only recently, however, have criteria been established which make certain agents practical for increasing plasma osmolarity. To adequately maintain a significant plasma:aqueous:vitreous osmotic gradient, certain criteria must be met:

1. The agent must have a low molecular weight—which will provide a greater osmotic effect since the number of molecules, not their weight, is what is important.
2. The agent must be nontoxic.
3. The agent must show poor ocular penetrance.

Sucrose and sorbitol will maintain an adequate gradient since they penetrate the eye poorly; but because of their high molecular weight, large doses are required, which makes them impractical. In addition, they may cause renal damage. On the other hand, sodium chloride is nontoxic and of low molecular weight; but it penetrates the eye rapidly.

Although these agents are relatively safe, the ophthalmologist should be familiar with their side effects:

1. Angina, arrhythmias, hypertension, congestive heart failure, pulmonary edema (associated with rapid expansion of blood volume)
2. Headache and back pain (due to reduced intracranial pressure)
3. More serious cerebral complications (e.g., subdural hematoma)
4. Diuresis with intravenous agents
5. Nausea and vomiting with oral agents
6. Specific complications related to an agent
   Slough—urea
   Hematuria and anuria—intravenous glycerin
   Gastric disorders and diarrhea—oral vitamin C
   Hyperglycemia—glycerin

I find oral glycerin (Osmoglyn, Alcon Labs, Inc., Milwaukee; Glyrol, Smith, Miller & Patch, New York City) to be the most convenient of all the agents. It can be given orally, is safe, and does not promote a diffuse diuresis. The incidence of nausea and vomiting is low, which I have attributed to serving the glycerin in cracked ice, not oversedating the patient, and having the patient in the supine position. I have used it in nearly every cataract extraction for more than eleven years.

In an experimental study[24] I found that I was able to achieve a lower intraocular pressure using glycerin preoperatively, along with retrobulbar anesthesia and 5 minutes of digital massage, than I could without the glycerin. Isosorbide (Hydronol, Atlas Chemical Industries, Inc., Wilmington, Delaware) may be substituted for glycerin. With a dose of 1.5 Gm/kg body weight, its pressure-lowering effect is similar to glycerin's. It appears to have certain advantages. It has no caloric value and is not metabolized. Thus it may be safer for diabetics. In addition, side effects such as nausea, vomiting, headache, and backache appear to be less frequent.

If the surgery is performed under general anesthesia, an intravenous preparation such as 20% mannitol (Osmitrol, Travenol Laboratories, Inc., Morton Grove, Illinois) or urea in the form of a 30% lyophilized solution (Urevert, Travenol Laboratories) may be used. The great drawback of urea is the serious consequence of extravasation at the needle site; mannitol is therefore preferred. An indwelling catheter may be necessary in some cases since the urine flow rate with mannitol is about five times greater than with glycerin.

Despite their drawbacks, all hyperosmotic agents are a useful adjunct to cataract surgery.

The mode of action of these agents is presumed to be removal of fluid from the vitreous, thereby reducing its volume. Although such a statement is difficult to prove, the following data justify the assumption: Bucci and Neuschüler[8] evaluated, by Jaeger's apparatus, the depth of the anterior chamber in humans after the oral administration of 50% glycerin in doses of 1 Gm/kg body weight. The mean deepening of the anterior chamber in normal eyes was 0.04 mm; in glaucomatous and cataractous eyes (unoperated) 0.05 mm; and in operated eyes 0.2 mm. From their study the dehydrating effect of glycerin would appear to be exerted on the vitreous, since only in this way can a deepening of the anterior chamber be explained.

The same authors[7] later noted that glycerin administered orally does not inhibit aqueous humor production (unlike acetazolamide) but, on the contrary, facilitates the fluid's passage into the anterior chamber at a given interval after administration. Bucci[6] had studied the effect of orally administered glycerin on the weight and volume of the vitreous body in rabbits and had obtained a constant reduction of the weight and volume of the vitreous. A surprisingly small decrease in volume such as 4% was sufficient to cause a profound drop in intraocular pressure. The removal of 0.12 ml of retrovitreal fluid (slightly greater than 2% of vitreous volume) produces a profound hypotony. This work was later corroborated by Robbins and Galin[37] using a similar technique.

Bucci and Virno[9] performed a dramatic experiment wherein they trephined a corneal button from rabbits' eyes and placed a piston attached to a series of levers on the lens. The piston fell as the rabbits were given a hyperosmotic agent. There was no fall in the control eyes, in which a hyperosmotic agent was not given. Presumably the posterior displacement of the lens was due to a reduction in vitreous volume.

POSTERIOR SCLEROTOMY. A posterior sclerotomy with drainage of vitreous fluid preparatory to cataract surgery is a seldom used but effective method of preventing operative loss of vitreous. This technique has been recommended by Iliff[23] when medical (hyperosmotic agents) or mechanical (digital massage) means have failed to achieve a tonometric scale reading of 10 units or more with a 5.5-gram weight.

A pars planotomy is performed in the upper temporal quadrant of the globe in the following manner: A flap of conjunctiva and Tenon's capsule is turned down from the upper fornix, exposing the sclera. A Hildreth or Scheie cautery needle is applied to the exposed sclera 6 mm from and parallel to the limbus until a slight shrinkage of tissue is noted over a 1 × 4 mm area. A narrow-bladed Graefe knife is then passed through this area of the sclera and pars plana and directed posteriorly and inferiorly toward the lower temporal quadrant of the globe to a depth of 1 cm, as marked with methylene blue on the blade of the knife. The point enters the temporal vitreous lake, which lies between the central formed vitreous and the temporal retina. The blade is turned, spreading the lips of the wound and creating a channel for drainage of fluid. When the eye is soft, the knife is withdrawn. The scleral incision does not need to be sutured. Iliff prefers the knife to aspiration with an 18-gauge needle because he considers the knife less traumatic.

I have modified the foregoing pars planotomy technique and find it to be a most useful and simple procedure in the rare instance when it is necessary. At a point 5 mm from the limbus in the superior temporal quadrant, a small conjunctival incision is made to expose the sclera, which is marked at this point. A 25- or 27-gauge Rizzuti-Spirizzi keratome cannula attached to a syringe is passed through the sclera and pars plana at this point and is directed superiorly and posteriorly—where the retrovitreal space is usually found. Aspiration pressure is exerted on the syringe as the cannula is passed through the vitreous. When the retrovitreal space is reached, a sudden gush of aqueous enters the syringe.

The globe will become mushy soft from aspiration of as little as 0.25 ml. These cannulas are perfectly suited for such a procedure (Fig. 4-27). They are so sharp they will pass through the sclera without fixation of the globe. No attempt is made to remove formed vitreous, merely retrovitreal aqueous. In fact, formed vitreous will not pass through this needle. A 25- or 27-gauge disposable needle attached to a syringe may be substituted because of its sharpness.

My view is that the technique should be reserved for the rare patient who cannot be given a hyperosmotic agent or who vomits the preparation—in whom the intraocular pressure cannot be reduced to hypotony and in whom vitreous was lost during surgery on the first eye. If a tonometric reading of 10 or more scale units (5.5-gram weight) cannot be achieved, a careful search for extraglobal pressure should be conducted. A faulty speculum, an everted upper tarsus with the use of lid sutures, a tight lateral canthus, inadequate akinesia, residual extraocular muscle activity, or a retrobulbar hemorrhage may be causing the high reading.

Reduction of external pressure on the vitreous. The advantage of reducing vitreous bulk, as described, is obvious since such a reduction will then require a greater force exerted against the vitreous to cause a rupture of the anterior hyaloid membrane. Nevertheless, minimizing these forces is of critical importance and is clearly the stamp of the skillful surgeon.

DIGITAL PRESSURE. The benefits of digital ocular compression in reducing orbital volume and thereby decreasing external pressure on the vitreous have been discussed.

Technique of separating the eyelids

The technique of separating the eyelids may very well be responsible for most of the inadequacies encountered in reducing external pressure on the vitreous. The variety of the methods of globe exposure is adequate testimony to the inefficacy of these methods. Proper exposure of the operative field is essential in all surgery. Several factors alter the degree of exposure in ophthalmic surgery—a deep-set eye, a short palpebral fissure, microphthalmos, a large globe (e.g., in high myopia), and an inadequate orbit as in some cases of exophthalmos.

The most effective method of avoiding pressure on the globe involves the use of separate upper and lower lid retractors, such as those recommended by Desmarres. This involves the use of a trained alert assistant throughout the entire procedure, however, and has detracted from the popularity of the technique.

Exposure must be obtained with the lids well away from the globe and the tarsus in its normal plane. If the tarsus has a rather large vertical dimension, its eversion may press more posteriorly on the globe and in a more perpendicular direction—a situation to be avoided. Lid sutures and small marginal lid clamps (Castroviejo) provide excellent exposure; but all too often the very dangers they seek to avoid are inherent in this method.

The lid speculum is convenient but has limitations. The main source of pressure is the weight of the central or screw end of the speculum, which is the most dependent part of the instrument and which exerts pressure on the lateral aspect of the globe. This pressure may be minimized somewhat by placing a cotton pledget between the screw end of the instrument and the skin surface of the lateral orbital margin. Some specula, such as the one-piece Colybri-Barraquer blepharostat, actually raise intraocular pressure to a dangerous level before the incision is made (Fig. 3-4). Many of the shortcomings of the speculum have been eliminated by the Guyton-Park and Maumenee-Park versions. The latter, however, do not permit different degrees of retraction for upper and lower eyelids.

I find separate upper and lower eyelid retractors[21] made of stainless steel wire most acceptable (Figs. 3-5 to 3-7). The curved end of the retractor fits be-

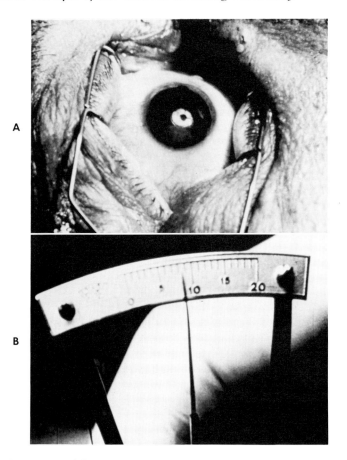

A

B

Fig. 3-4. **A,** One-piece Colybri-Barraquer blepharostat. **B,** Intraocular pressure is 10.2 mm Schiøtz. (From Jaffe, N. S.: Cataract surgery and its complications, St. Louis, 1972, The C. V. Mosby Co.)

hind the tarsus and is sufficiently broad to eliminate the notch type of retraction that occurs with single lid sutures. The curved end is approximately the same length as the tarsus, thereby eliminating any bending or folding of the tarsus. The retraction is in the direct plane of action of the lids. There is no pressure on the globe, and the exposure exceeds that of the speculum and eyelid sutures. A no. 1 nylon suture is tied to the end of the retractor and clamped to the drapes; thus no assistance is required for exposure. There are no annoying screws or locks to contend with; the retractors are easily and readily removed. These retractors permit different degrees of retraction of the upper and lower eyelids. When excessive retraction raises intraocular pressure, the lower eyelid is retracted less so exposure of the globe above need not be compromised.

Satisfactory anesthesia and akinesia. Residual extraocular or orbicularis muscle activity may exert significant pressure on the globe. If ocular movements persist after retrobulbar injection, the injection may be repeated or the individual rectus muscles may be injected directly.

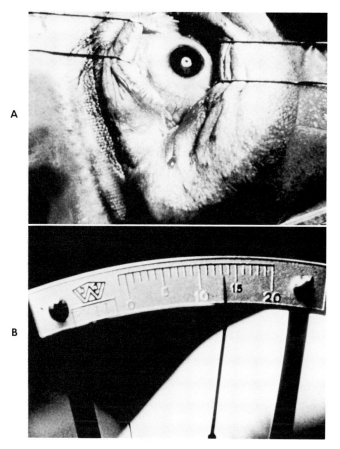

Fig. 3-5. **A,** Separate upper and lower eyelid Jaffe retractors placed in the same eye as in Fig. 3-4, immediately after the Colybri-Barraquer blepharostat was removed. **B,** Intraocular pressure is 4.0 mm Schiøtz. (From Jaffe, N. S.: Cataract surgery and its complications, St. Louis, 1972, The C. V. Mosby Co.)

The technique of performing the retrobulbar injection is important to avoid a retrobulbar hemorrhage. A blunt-tipped needle may be used but is probably not necessary if the fluid is slowly injected as soon as the needle penetrates the skin. Slow injection ensures against perforation of large vessels and the optic nerve. The volume of injected fluid should be small (2 to 3 ml), especially with a shallow orbit, tight lids, or a proptotic globe.

A significant retrobulbar hemorrhage is easy to detect; but a smaller hemorrhage may present few signs. A stainless steel autoclavable tonometer is indispensable in this regard and should be available on the instrument stand.

Avoidance of complications

Just as it takes only a small decrease in vitreous volume to cause a profound hypotony, so it requires only a minor extraocular force to displace the vitreous. An elevation of intraocular pressure may be readily detected by using the

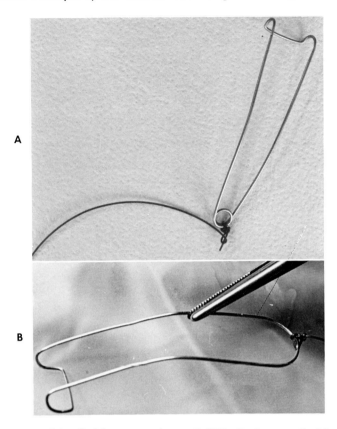

Fig. 3-6. **A,** New-model Jaffe lid retractor (Storz E-997). **B,** Givner-Jaffe lid retractor (Storz E-996). No. 0 nylon suture tied to the end of the retractor. The suture is clamped to drape sheets with a hemostat and may be autoclaved. (From Jaffe, N. S.: Cataract surgery and its complications, St. Louis, 1972, The C. V. Mosby Co.)

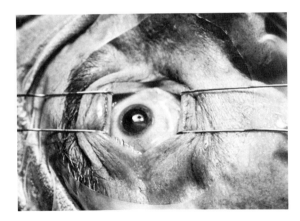

Fig. 3-7. Retraction of eyelids in their direct plane of action. The eyelids make no contact with the globe and there are no annoying screws or locks on the retractors. (From Jaffe, N. S.: Cataract surgery and its complications, St. Louis, 1972, The C. V. Mosby Co.)

tonometer. Continued digital massage will often cause a lowering of the pressure to safe levels after minor retrobulbar bleeding, but a significant hemorrhage should result in postponement of surgery.

Serous or hemorrhagic choroidal detachment. Serous or hemorrhagic choroidal detachment probably occurs in every decompression procedure performed on the eye. It appears as a dark, curved, elevated line with the convexity toward the disc. It is peripheral and found mostly in the inferior quadrants. The resulting mass may create a force sufficient to compress the vitreous to a dangerous degree. There are three forces to be considered in its pathogenesis:

1. The first is the *intraocular pressure*, which tends to prevent transudation from the choroidal vessels. This, of course, falls to 0 as soon as the globe is opened.

2. The second is the *intravascular pressure*. Since transudation occurs chiefly at the capillary level, the blood pressure within the choroidal capillaries is considered. According to Best and Taylor[4] the blood pressure at the arterial end is about 32 mm and at the venous end 12 mm. This force favors transudation into the tissue fluids.

3. Offsetting the intravascular pressure is the third force, the *oncotic pressure*, exerted by the protein colloids of the plasma, which tends to draw fluids from the tissues into the vascular tree.

A most important consideration may be how long the globe remains open. Possibly the longer the choroidal vessels are exposed to an intraocular pressure of 0, the greater is the likelihood of choroidal detachment.

We can only speculate on the role played by the transudate in compressing the vitreous at surgery. In considering all the forces that come into play on opening the globe, we may wonder whether any measures can be adopted to minimize vitreous compression. A precipitous fall in intraocular pressure favors more massive transudation. The fall may be largely avoided by reducing the intraocular pressure to hypotony before making the incision.

A rare but dangerous phenomenon is the sudden occurrence of a massive serous choroidal detachment. This is illustrated in the following case: A 74-year-old woman had a cataract removed from her right eye without complication. The anterior face of the vitreous appeared concave, and there was not the least sign of a vitreous bulge. Suddenly the vitreous began to push forward. A large choroidal detachment appeared in the superior temporal quadrant. It was dome-shaped and presented more than two thirds the way across the pupil. Formed vitreous escaped from the eye. A hasty diagnosis of expulsive hemorrhage was made. The emergency suture was tied at 12 o'clock. A subchoroidal tap was performed in the region of the detachment. A clear slightly yellow fluid escaped. Finally, a partial anterior vitrectomy was performed when there was no further progression of the choroidal effusion. Ruiz and Salmonsen[39] have described two similar cases. They call this entity "expulsive choroidal effusion."

Collapse of the sclera. Collapse of the sclera may create a force sufficient to compress the vitreous, with subsequent loss of vitreous during cataract surgery. It is probably one of the commonest causes of operative loss of vitreous and is usually undiagnosed. Although Flieringa[17] is largely credited with the technique of scleral fixation, van der Hoeve[46] in 1919 recommended the use of four episcleral sutures placed between the limbus and the insertion of the rectus muscles. If the pull on these sutures by the assistant is too great, however, the diminution of the surface will become considerable and the contents of the globe may be displaced.

Flieringa designed a ring made of stainless steel with a thickness of 0.3 mm and a diameter of 20 mm. He applied this to be concentric to the cornea. With the assumption that the eyeball is of normal size, the distance between the ring and the limbus will be 5 mm; in a larger eyeball a ring of 22 mm will be needed. The ring is fastened in the following manner: The conjunctiva is incised and the sclera exposed in eight places equally distributed on the total circumference. At these eight points the suture is brought through the episclera and the ring is thus firmly attached to the sclera. Alternate sutures are cut off close to the knot; the others are kept long. By accurate traction on these sutures, the tendency to scleral collapse and displacement of intraocular contents can be greatly reduced.

There have been variations and modifications of the Flieringa ring—notably the double ring of Legrand[5] (consisting of a smaller ring above a larger ring and available in two sizes, 14 × 23 mm and 17 × 24 mm) and the rings of

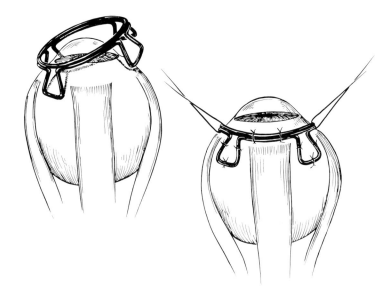

Fig. 3-8. The scleral expander is composed of a ring with four malleable wings that can be adjusted to the size of the globe. After peritomy and exposure of the muscles, the expander is best inserted by placing the lower wings on each side of the inferior rectus, inferiorly, and then inserting the upper wings superiorly. (From Girard, L. J.: In Emery, J., and Paton, D., editors: Current concepts in cataract surgery: selected proceedings of the Third Biennial Cataract Surgical Congress, St. Louis, 1974, The C. V. Mosby Co.)

Neubauer and of Mackensen. Girard[20] has designed a scleral expander for the prevention of scleral collapse during intraocular surgery. It is the most complex and cumbersome of all these instruments, but probably the most effective (Fig. 3-8).

Flieringa[17] recommends his perilimbal ring in the following situations: cataract extraction in high myopes, all cataracts in which one suspects a fluid vitreous, the discission of secondary cataracts as well as inflammatory pupillary membranes, the extraction of dislocated lenses, surgery for iris cysts, and penetrating keratoplasties exceeding 5 mm. Other men, however, consider the indications to be more limited.

Probably the greatest usefulness of the Flieringa ring is in linear extractions, which are usually performed in very young individuals. In these the sclera is highly elastic and collapses easily when the globe is decompressed, producing a marked forward propulsion of the lens-iris diaphragm immediately on entrance into the globe.

Mechanical factors. Mechanical factors that cause pressure on the vitreous

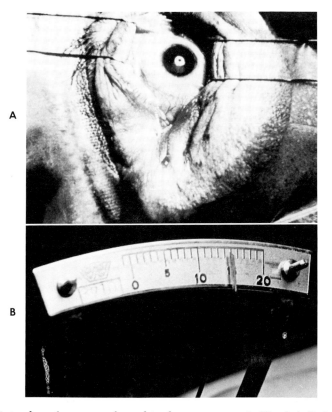

Fig. 3-9. A, Lateral canthotomy performed in the same eye as in Fig. 3-4. B, Intraocular pressure less than 3.0 mm Schiøtz. (From Jaffe, N. S.: Cataract surgery and its complications, St. Louis, 1972, The C. V. Mosby Co.)

include orbital abnormalities (e.g., oxycephaly), orbital masses (neoplasms or hyperplasias associated with endocrine exophthalmos), abnormalities of the eyelids (shortening of the palpebral fissure), and abnormalities of the conjunctiva (essential shrinkage). There is probably no satisfactory method of managing these problems. It is safe to make use of a liberal lateral canthotomy (Fig. 3-9). In exophthalmos with increased orbital resistance, it may be advisable to eliminate the speculum or lid sutures and merely resort to a superior rectus bridle suture for exposure. If eyelid retraction causes the shrunken conjunctiva to press on the globe, the conjunctiva may be incised. The availability of a tonometer is invaluable. If the intraocular pressure cannot be reduced to a safe surgical level, one should consider a preliminary posterior sclerotomy, as previously suggested. In these cases the ingenuity of the surgeon is tested most severely.

The surgeon should be on guard at all times for the development of vitreous loss during cataract surgery. I have found the following five situations especially dangerous:

1. Young patient. Digital pressure and hyperosmotic agents cause little reduction in vitreous volume probably because there is little free or nonlinked water in the vitreous and these eyes also show a marked tendency to scleral collapse.

2. Eyes with a shallow anterior chamber and narrow angle. Digital pressure may completely occlude the angle and create a misdirected flow of aqueous into the vitreous. The intraocular pressure rises rather than falls as digital pressure is performed. A preliminary posterior sclerotomy is useful in this situation.

3. Previous peripheral iridectomy. These eyes often show a forward displacement of the lens-iris-vitreous diaphragm. The iris may prolapse as soon as the incision is made.

4. Certain anatomic factors—short thick neck, proptosis, etc. The patient's head should be propped up to prevent hyperextension of the neck.

5. Evidence or positive history of operative loss of vitreous in the opposite eye. Prolonged digital pressure and a hyperosmotic agent should be used. Posterior sclerotomy may be performed if the intraocular pressure does not fall to a safe level.

During surgery

Sometimes, despite the precautions previously outlined or when the likelihood of vitreous loss was not appreciated beforehand, a dangerous situation becomes apparent immediately after surgical decompression of the globe. The signs of such impending danger may be so obvious as to be recognized by even an inexperienced surgeon; or the signs may be more subtle and recognizable only with experience.

One sign of increased vitreous pressure is forward displacement of the lens

and iris with gaping of the wound. This situation may complicate the enlargement of the incision since placing the blades of the scissors between the cornea
and the bulging iris becomes increasingly difficult. The iris may actually prolapse.

Another important sign is the appearance of horizontal lines of tension or
creases in the cornea. If the vitreous pressure is low, a vertical or circular
indentation of the cornea will appear after the incision is made. The presence
of *horizontal* creases, however, is a dangerous sign because conjunctival ecchy-
mosis, increasing in degree, often signals a retrobulbar hemorrhage or a
"retrobulbar" injection outside Tenon's capsule.

The causes of this critical situation are often not immediately apparent.
They are usually related to some form of external pressure exerted against
the vitreous.

1. The method of lid retraction may be faulty.
2. There may be inadequate exposure and pressure against the globe because of a tight lateral canthus.
3. There may be residual ocular movements and some residual orbicularis
   oculi function.
4. There may be inadequate oxygenation of the patient or a high degree
   of restlessness.
5. There may be scleral collapse, especially in young patients, although
   this occurs in older individuals more often than is generally appreciated.
6. A significant retrobulbar hemorrhage may be present.
7. A subchoroidal hemorrhage or serous effusion may exert pressure on
   the vitreous.

The surgeon should make every attempt to determine the cause of the increased vitreous pressure. Retraction of the lower lid should be terminated by
releasing the lower blade of the speculum, loosening the lower lid suture, or
removing the independent lower lid retractor. Sometimes these measures cause
less wound gape. If it has not already been done, a lateral canthotomy should
be performed. The corneoscleral incision may be held closed for several minutes
and mild pressure exerted against the cornea with a scalpel handle. If the
wound gapes again when the cornea is retracted, the situation has not been
remedied.

The following procedure, though not always simple to perform, may be
useful for remedying recurrent wound gape:

The wound should be closed by drawing up the preplaced sutures. A
bubble of air is placed in the anterior chamber; it will often escape if the
vitreous is under great pressure, in which case a surgeon's knot should be made
with each suture, if air continues to escape from the anterior chamber, addi
tional sutures should be inserted and a single tie placed in each. Air will
usually be retained at this juncture, and the lens-iris diaphragm is forced posteriorly.

Once the lens-iris diaphragm is in place, there is no need to rush. The sclera is exposed in the superior temporal quadrant. A 25- or 27-gauge Rizzuti-Spirizzi cannula needle attached to a syringe is inserted through the sclera at a point 5 mm from the limbus. The instrument is so sharp that pressure exerted against the globe during its insertion is minimal. It is directed superoposteriorly until the retrovitreal space is entered, at which point fluid may be aspirated into the syringe. The cornea will then show a vertical oval fold, indicating lowered intravitreal pressure. The sutures are untied and the wound reopened. The cataract extraction may then proceed in the usual manner. Many times, the impending vitreous loss will be averted by this procedure.

A Flieringa ring may be applied after the posterior sclerotomy is performed to minimize the effect of scleral collapse if it is a cause of vitreous bulge.

By indirect ophthalmoscopy the surgeon can detect whether the vitreous has been pushed forward by a subchoroidal hemorrhage; a dark choroidal mass will become evident in the fundus. If blood bursts through the choroid and retina, an expulsive hemorrhage has occurred.

MANAGEMENT OF OPERATIVE LOSS OF VITREOUS

No matter how skillful the surgeon or how astute his judgment, operative loss of vitreous will occur. There has been a gradual departure from the early tendency to simply close the wound with as little loss of formed vitreous as possible. Numerous methods of managing operative loss of vitreous now exist, some of which appear to be contradictory.

Vitreous replacement

Vitreous replacement has been advocated in massive losses of vitreous. Some authors extol the benefits of vitreous replacement, whereas others consider it entirely unnecessary. The former are motivated by the fear of an immediate intraocular hemorrhage, later retinal detachment, or even phthisis bulbi.

As early as 1883, Andrews[1] successfully treated posttraumatic collapse of the globe with injections of sterile saline solution; and Starr[42] later did the same. Knapp[27] expanded the indications by recommending the injection of lukewarm sterile saline solution in profound postoperative hypotony and in massive loss of fluid vitreous, especially after a bulbar collapse associated with a perforating wound. In the last he felt that the injected saline not only accomplished a refilling of the globe but also served to inhibit inflammation.

In 1916 Mayweg[31] stated that vitreous lost in small amount is spontaneously replaced, but in massive vitreous loss saline replacement is the surest way to avoid phthisis bulbi. In the same year, however, Schreiber[40] performed experiments on rabbits and observed that the removal of vitreous, even in large amounts, was followed by a spontaneous refilling of the vitreous cavity. He related this to his clinical observations that postoperative and posttraumatic massive loss of vitreous is usually followed by a spontaneous refilling. He stated that even if the procedure is well tolerated it merely adds a supplementary trauma. If the collapse persists for 2 or 3 days, however, a saline injection then may be of value.

There is no valid statistical series relating to the benefits of saline injection as opposed to permitting spontaneous refilling of the globe. Thus there is little to be gained by reviewing the numerous reports on this subject. With the advent of modern cataract surgery, including better methods of wound closure, less is to be feared from bulbar collapse once the risk of immediate intraocular hemorrhage has passed. Recently a long list of vitreous substitutes has become available.

Ice cold water

Ice cold water poured on the prolapsed vitreous to provoke its retraction has been recommended by Moutinho and Brégeat.[33]

Gas refrigerants

Gas refrigerants such as tetrafluorodichloroethane (Freon) have been advocated by Miller and his colleagues[32] to cause vitreous retraction, although Magdalena[28] attributes the benefits obtained to choroidal vasoconstriction.

Reduction of prolapsed vitreous without resection

Castroviejo[10] first closes the wound with an adequate number of corneoscleral sutures. He then engages the prolapsed or incarcerated vitreous by passing a specially designed cyclodialysis spatula (15 mm long, 0.75 mm wide) through the temporal extremity of the wound. The vitreous is drawn inferiorly by a sweep made parallel to the plane of the iris. This is repeated until there is no vitreous in the wound. The anterior chamber is filled with air, and the pupil constricted with a miotic.

I have personally been less fortunate than Castroviejo in utilizing this procedure. Too often, I find vitreous regaining access to the wound, with subsequent distortion of the pupil.

Maumenee[29] in 1957 advocated a similar technique in which he leaves his most temporal suture untied, inserts a tightly wound cotton stick applicator into the anterior chamber through this opening, engages the prolapsed vitreous, draws it out of the wound, and resects it.

Removal of fluid vitreous

In 1965, Maumenee[30] advocated an excellent method of reducing prolapsed vitreous that enables the wound to be sutured without vitreous between its lips and air to be placed in the anterior chamber. An 18-gauge needle that has had the tip filed off and is marked 1.5 cm from its tip is inserted into the vitreous for about a centimeter. Gentle traction is then placed on a 2 ml syringe attached to the needle. As soon as the pocket of fluid vitreous is tapped, 1 to 2 ml may be aspirated. Formed vitreous in the anterior chamber will then retract.

Management of the iris

When the vitreous face ruptures, sometimes not all the vitreous can be swept back into the pupillary space. The iris is thrown into folds. It may even roll posteriorly and be lost from view. Within a few days these folds become so fibrosed that they cannot be unfolded even with a forceps. For this reason a large sector iridectomy has been practiced and may be combined with an inferior sphincterotomy to avoid an updrawn pupil. Castroviejo,[11] however, and Barraquer and co-workers[3] recommend maintenance of the round pupil.

Resection has probably been the most frequently practiced procedure for operative loss of vitreous. Classically resection has been performed after the wound is closed by pulling up the preplaced corneoscleral sutures. All vitreous that persists between the lips of the wound is resected. A spatula is used to ensure that no residual vitreous remains incarcerated between the lips of the wound. Air is then placed in the anterior chamber. I have used this technique with less than ideal results. The residual vitreous readheres to the wound and causes marked distortion of the iris with displacement of the pupil. Frequently the air penetrates the disrupted vitreous and lodges in the center of the globe.

Partial anterior vitrectomy

The technique of partial anterior vitrectomy has gained popularity in recent years. Because of several obvious advantages that make it the management procedure of choice in operative loss of vitreous, I have been using it for several years.

The term *partial* signifies that the entire anterior portion of the vitreous is not resected—in fact, the part attached to the pars plana and ora (vitreous base) is left intact. Therefore partial anterior vitrectomy is a more suitable term than anterior vitrectomy.

Credit for the technique correctly belongs to Kasner,[25] who has employed it since 1961. His first experience involved a boy whose eye was lacerated open along the horizontal axis. Traumatic aniridia and aphakia were present and most of the vitreous had been avulsed; some of it was actually present on the boy's face. He appeared anophthalmic on lid closure. He was taken to the operating room, where the remainder of the vitreous was removed as close as possible to the retina. The wound was tightly closed with sutures, and the globe filled with air and saline solution. The eye recovered remarkably, and visual acuity seven years later was 20/50 with a contact lens. The retina is now normal, and the vitreous cavity appears optically empty.

This experience, combined with subsequent examples, teaches us that an eye can survive remarkably well without vitreous—which should come as no surprise since, in the natural course of senescence, liquefaction of the vitreous gel occurs and greatly reduces the formed elements. In myopic eyes and other pathologic and posttraumatic states, it is not unusual to find a vitreous cavity that appears optically empty because of conversion of the gel to a completely fluid state.

Anterior vitrectomy treats the vitreous as if it were a vestigial organ (e.g., the appendix). Kasner[25] considers the vitreous as the "enemy." When it causes trouble, he gets rid of it. If many of the complications resulting from operative

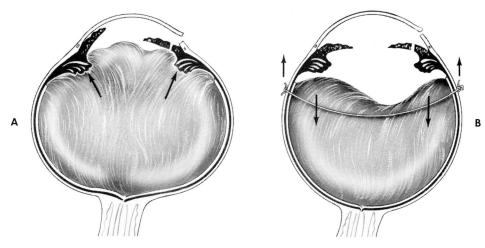

Fig. 3-10. **A,** Collapse of the globe after operative loss of vitreous. The angle of the anterior chamber is closed by the iris, which is pushed up from below. **B,** Application of a Flieringa ring maintains the shape of the globe. The iris tends to fall back posteriorly as vitreous is removed, thus keeping the angle open at all times. (From Jaffe, N. S.: Cataract surgery and its complications, St. Louis, 1972, The C. V. Mosby Co.)

loss of vitreous are due to direct contact of the vitreous with other structures, incarceration of the vitreous into the operative wound, fibroplasia of the residual vitreous, and inflammation, then the prudent course would appear to be to rid the anterior segment of the eye of vitreous before these changes can take place. All previous methods, no matter how expertly applied, usually fail in this regard.

In children, in whom scleral collapse usually occurs, a scleral ring may be applied before the vitrectomy is begun. A scleral ring may be of advantage too in adults, though not always an absolute necessity. The wound should be closed by drawing up the preplaced sutures and tying them with a surgeon's knot—which also will facilitate placement of the scleral ring. The beneficial effect of the ring is attributable to the fact that when the globe collapses the angle is often closed by iris pushed up from below (Fig. 3-10). This pushing up is caused by the circumferential residuum of vitreous just under the peripheral portion of iris at the vitreous base.

It is remarkable how quickly the vitreous over the iris and lips of the wound becomes fibrinous. Iris contracture pulls the periphery of the iris up against the cornea, thus making it difficult to rid the angle of vitreous. The result is usually an angle that becomes permanently closed in many areas. If the ring is applied first, the shape of the globe is maintained. The iris tends to fall back posteriorly as vitreous is removed, thus keeping the angle open at all times.

Once the ring is securely in place (four episcleral sutures instead of the customary eight are usually adequate), the wound is reopened. The incision is enlarged to 200° to facilitate vitreous removal and avoid damage to the corneal endothelium. The cornea is retracted by the assistant and the vitrectomy is performed by the open sky technique.

Chunks of vitreous are picked up with a cellulose sponge (e.g. Weck-Cell, E. Weck & Co., Long Island City, New York). They are cut at the pupillary plane by scissors (Fig. 4-10). They should not be pulled outside the globe to be cut since they may, if stretched to excess, cause a retinal detachment or a vitreous hemorrhage. I prefer to use long-bladed scissors at first and then change to short-bladed scissors such as those of de Wecker or Barraquer when smaller bundles of vitreous are excised from the face of the iris or from the angle. This procedure is tedious since it must be performed meticulously to be effective.

After a moderate amount of vitreous is removed from the pupillary area, the iris will fall posteriorly—exposing the angle. Small triangular bits of the cellulose sponge are then applied to the surface of the iris and the angle to remove the remaining vitreous from the anterior chamber. The sponge will often swell because of absorption of fluid, but it will usually retain its contact with formed vitreous so the vitreous can be cut.

When vitreous can no longer be picked up at the temporal and nasal extremities of the incision, the anterior chamber is free of vitreous. Additional vitreous should then be removed from the pupillary space. Cellulose sponges which are long and narrow (2 × 8 mm) are presently available and are very useful for picking up vitreous in the pupillary axis behind the level of the iris. This can be done with minimal iris contact and results in much less postoperative iritis.

Finally, the pupil is constricted with acetylcholine. If the pupil is round, its shape should be retained since this will aid in preventing later incarceration of vitreous in the wound. The anterior chamber should be filled with air or balanced salt solution to facilitate suturing.

It is especially important that wound closure be meticulous. A subconjunctival injection of a long-acting steroid should be made.

When properly performed, a partial anterior vitrectomy empties the entire anterior chamber and the anterior third of the vitreous cavity of formed vitreous (Fig. 3-11). Because of the associated intraocular inflammation, local as well as systemic steroids should be prescribed. An injection of 1 ml of a long-acting steroid at weekly intervals under Tenon's capsule may be given if necessary.

Although I have not found it necessary, Gass[19] prefers to aspirate fluid vitreous before the vitrectomy according to the technique suggested by Maumenee. Such aspiration causes the formed vitreous to retract and perhaps facilitates removal of vitreous from the angle. There may be a tendency, however, to remove less vitreous. Also the maneuver may delude the surgeon into thinking an adequate anterior vitrectomy has been performed since the iris falls back when the retrovitreal fluid is aspirated. The pocket may refill after the incision is closed, and formed vitreous may fill the anterior chamber; but if we keep this possibility in mind, a combination of the two procedures may be useful since the time required for the surgery may be shortened and perhaps the performance facilitated.

Cerasoli[12] studied a serious of partial anterior vitrectomies, according to the

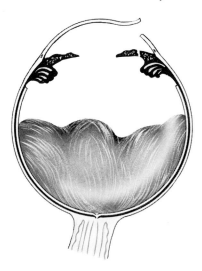

Fig. 3-11. When properly performed, a partial anterior vitrectomy empties the entire chamber and the anterior third of the vitreous cavity of formed vitreous. (From Jaffe, N. S.: Cataract surgery and its complications, St. Louis, 1972, The C. V. Mosby Co.)

technique of Kasner,[25] performed for operative loss of vitreous at the Bascom Palmer Eye Institute. In the series seventeen of the eighteen eyes were white quiet eyes, and only one had cells in the anterior chamber. Twenty-eight percent showed macular lesions; 6% had corneal complications. There were nine peaked pupils and nine unpeaked pupils. Nine had vitreous attached to the surgical wound—three in the form of a sheet, two with thick strands, and four with thin strands. Seven eyes had vitreous at or posterior to the plane of the iris; eleven had vitreous in the anterior chamber. The fundus was normal in twelve eyes, abnormal in six. Of the latter, two had cystoid macular edema, one had cystoid macular edema with macular pucker, one had macular pucker, one had atrophy of the pigment epithelium at the posterior pole, and one had a pigmented scar temporal to the macula.

When properly performed, the technique produces esthetic results that speak for themselves (Fig. 3-12). If the pupil is round, it will remain so and the peripheral iris openings will remain patent. If a sector iridectomy has been performed, there will be no tendency for the inferior pupillary edge to migrate upward.

Although our surgical instinct might react favorably to the technique of partial anterior vitrectomy, it is possible that a large series with long-term follow-up will reveal serious complications—e.g., vitreous hemorrhage, persistent iritis, persistent cystoid macular edema, retinal detachment.

Some authors report more favorable results; but I prefer to remain cautious, since I have observed retinal detachments in two patients and have knowledge of others and I have observed vitreous hemorrhage in three patients. Nevertheless, I feel that a partial anterior vitrectomy is the best way to manage operative

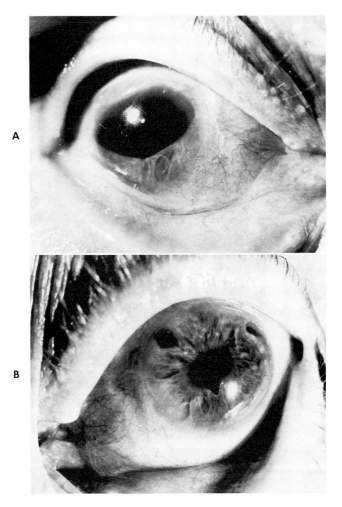

Fig. 3-12. This patient had cataract surgery in both eyes six years apart. In each instance there was loss of formed vitreous. **A,** In the first eye the vitreous was swept back into the anterior chamber, and the chamber was filled with air. A sector iridectomy was not performed. Note the marked distortion of the pupil. Residual astigmatic error is 4.50 D. Cystoid macular edema was present for two years and was followed by some residual degeneration of the macula. Corrected visual acuity is 20/60. **B,** The second eye was managed by anterior vitrectomy. All the formed vitreous was removed from the anterior chamber. A small inferior sphincterotomy was performed. Note the patency of the peripheral iridotomies and the lack of distortion of the pupil. Residual astigmatic error is 0.75 D. Corrected visual acuity two years after surgery is 20/25. (From Jaffe, N. S.: The vitreous in clinical ophthalmology, St. Louis, 1969, The C. V. Mosby Co.)

loss of vitreous. The procedure must be correctly performed to avoid some of the complications seen earlier. *It is most important to cut the vitreous at the level of or slightly behind the iris to avoid excessive traction on the retina and its blood vessels.*

REFERENCES

1. Andrews, J. A.: On the injection of a weak sterile solution of sodium chloride into collapsed eyes, Arch. Ophthalmol. **29**:50, 1900.
2. Atkinson, W. S.: Local anesthesia in ophthalmology, Trans. Am. Ophthalmol. Soc. **32**:399, 1934.
3. Barraquer, J., Troutman, R. C., and Rutllán, J.: Surgery of the anterior segment of the eye, New York, 1964, McGraw-Hill Book Co.
4. Best, C. H., and Taylor, N. B.: The physiological basis of medical practice, ed. 3, Baltimore, 1943, The Williams & Wilkins Co.
5. Brini, A., Bronner, A., Gerhard, J. P., and Nordmann, J.: Biologie et chirurgie du corps vitré, Paris, 1968, Masson & Cie., Editeurs.
6. Bucci, M. G.: Modificazioni ponderali del vitreo di coniglio dopo somministrazione orale di glicerolo, Boll. Oculist. **42**:569, 1963.
7. Bucci, M. G., and Neuschüler, R.: Comportamento della profondità della camera anteriore dopo somministrazione di glicerolo per os, Boll. Oculist. **46**:116, 1967.
8. Bucci, M. G., and Neuschüler, R.: Indagini sul meccanismo d'azione ipotensiva oculare del glicerolo, Boll. Oculist. **42**:299, 1963.
9. Bucci, M. G., and Virno, M.: Azione disidratante delle sostanze osmotiche sui tessuti oculari di coniglio, Boll. Oculist. **47**:407, 1968.
10. Castroviejo, R.: Cataract surgery: the handling of complications, Am. J. Ophthalmol. **58**:68, 1964.
11. Castroviejo, R.: Handling of eyes with vitreous prolapse following cataract extraction, Am. J. Ophthalmol. **48**:397, 1959.
12. Cerasoli, J.: The (Kasner) technique of radial anterior vitrectomy in vitreous loss (a 30 case follow-up). In Welsh, R. C., and Welsh, J., editors: The new report on cataract surgery, Miami, 1969, Miami Educational Press.
13. Costomiris, G. A.: Du massage oculaire au point de vue historique et thérapeutique, et surtout du massage direct de la conjonctive de la cornée, Arch. Ophthalmol. **10**:37, 1890.
14. Curtin, B.: Tonometer compression as an efficient alternative to preoperative ocular massage, Am. J. Ophthalmol. **76**:472, 1973.
15. Donders, F. C.: Note in Zehender's Monatsblaetter, p. 302, 1872.
16. Dunphy, E. B.: Loss of vitreous in cataract extraction, J.A.M.A. **89**:2254, 1927.
17. Flieringa, H. J.: Procedure to prevent vitreous loss, Am. J. Ophthalmol. **36**:1618, 1953.
18. François, J., Gdal-On, M., Takeuchi, T., and Victoria-Troncoso, V.: Ocular hypotension and massage of the eyeball, Ann. Ophthalmol. **5**:645, 1973.
19. Gass, J. D. M.: Management of vitreous loss after cataract extraction, Arch. Ophthalmol. **83**:319, 1970.
20. Girard, L. J.: Use of the scleral expander in intraocular surgery. In Emery, J., and Paton, D., editors: Current concepts in cataract surgery: selected proceedings of the Third Biennial Cataract Surgical Congress, St. Louis, 1974, The C. V. Mosby Co.
21. Givner, I., Jaffe, N. S., and Teschner, B. M.: A lid retractor for cataract surgery, Am. J. Ophthalmol. **34**:108, 1954.
22. Hildreth, H. R.: Digital ocular compression preceding cataract surgery, Am. J. Ophthalmol. **51**:1237, 1961.
23. Iliff, C. E.: A surgically soft eye by posterior sclerotomy, Am. J. Ophthalmol. **61**:276, 1966.
24. Jaffe, N. S., and Light, D. S.: Oral glycerin in cataract surgery, Arch. Ophthalmol. **73**:516, 1965.
25. Kasner, D.: The technique of radial anterior vitrectomy in vitreous loss. In Welsh, R. C., and Welsh, J., editors: The new report on cataract surgery, Miami, 1969, Miami Educational Press.
26. Kirsch, R. E., and Steinman, W.: Digital pressure, an important safeguard in cataract surgery, Arch. Ophthalmol. **54**:697, 1955.
27. Knapp, H.: On the injection of a weak sterile salt solution into collapsed eyes, Arch. Ophthalmol. **28**:308, 1899.
28. Magdalena C. J.: Profilaxis mediante el frio, de las pérdidas de vitreo en la operación de catarata, Arch. Soc. Oftalmol. Hispanoam. **25**:253, 1965.
29. Maumenee, A. E.: Symposium: Postop-

erative cataract complications. III, Epithelial invasion of the anterior chamber; retinal detachment; corneal edema; anterior chamber hemorrhages, changes in the macula, Trans. Am. Acad. Ophthalmol. Otolaryngol. **61**:51, 1957.

30. Maumenee, A. E.: Cited by Vail, D.: After results of vitreous loss, Am. J. Ophthalmol. **59**:573, 1965.
31. Mayweg: Discussion of paper by Schreiber, L.: Ber. Dtsch. Ophthalmol. Ges. **40**:456, 1916.
32. Miller, H. A., Perdriel, G., Graveline, J., and Manent, P.: Note préliminaire sur l'utilisation de gaz réfrigerants en chirurgie oculaire, Bull. Soc. Ophtalmol. Fr. **64**:358, 1964.
33. Moutinho, H.: Discussion of paper by Sédan, J., Farnarier, G., and Brégeat, P.: Les ectopies cristalliniennes; indications et techniques chirurgicales, Ann. Ther. Clin. Ophtalmol. **16**:210, 1965.
34. Pagenstecher, H.: Ueber die Massage des Auges und deren Andwendung bei verschiedenen Augenerkrankungen, Zentralbl. Prakt. Augenheilkd. **2**:281, 1878.
35. Quinn, L. H., and Porter, J. C.: The removal of tritiated water from the vitreous of the dog, Trans. Am. Ophthalmol. Soc. **61**:181, 1963.
36. Richter, A. G.: A treatise on the extraction of the cataract. Translated from the German with a plate and notes by the translator, London, 1791, J. Murray.

37. Robbins, R., and Galin, M. A.: Effect of osmotic agents on the vitreous body, Arch. Ophthalmol. **82**:694, 1969.
38. Robbins, R., Blumenthal, M., and Galin, M. A.: Reduction of vitreous weight by ocular massage, Am. J. Ophthalmol. **69**:603, 1970.
39. Ruiz, R. S., and Salmonsen, P. C.: Expulsive choroidal effusion: A complication of intraocular surgery, Arch. Ophthalmol. (To be published.)
40. Schreiber, L.: Ueber Glaskörperverlust und spontanen Glaskörperersatz, Ber. Dtsch. Ophthalmol. Ges. **40**:456, 1916.
41. Smith, H.: The treatment of cataract, Calcutta, 1910, Thacker, Spink & Co.
42. Starr, E. G. On the injection of sterile salt solution into collapsed eyeballs. Report of two cases, Arch. Ophthalmol. **30**:418, 1901.
43. Vail, D.: After results of vitreous loss, Am. J. Ophthalmol. **59**:573, 1965.
44. Vail, D. T.: Loss of vitreous during cataract surgery, Highlights Ophthalmol. **11**:107, 1968.
45. Vail, D. T.: Lantern demonstration of the unmodified "Smith" operation for cataract, Ophthalmoscope **9**:232, 1911.
46. van der Hoeve, J.: Ein Verfahren zur Vorbengung von Glaskörpervorfall, Klin. Monatsbl. Augenheilkd. **62**:791, 1919.

4

Postoperative cataract complications related to the vitreous

NORMAN S. JAFFE

CYSTOID MACULAR EDEMA (IRVINE-GASS SYNDROME)

We have known for some time that macular edema may occur during the postoperative period of a cataract extraction. In 1952 Irvine[18] described a syndrome now bearing his name which included improvement of vision after cataract surgery followed by diminution of vision associated with a postoperative rupture of the anterior hyaloid membrane, with or without adherence of vitreous to the surgical wound.

Clinical findings

Although nearly twenty years have elapsed since Irvine described this postoperative cataract syndrome, the mechanism involved in its production has only recently come into sharper focus. Still some controversy surrounds this mechanism.

Irvine[18] postulated that the cause of the visual disturbance was either remote vitreous traction at the macula, initiated by adherence of vitreous to the operative wound, or viterous opacities associated with iritis. Since techniques and instrumentation for biomicroscopic examination of the posterior vitreous were not well advanced at that time, he was unable to accurately define the pathologic picture. Years later the role of vitreous traction was strongly implicated by some authors[28,32] but denied by others.[8,22,25] Painstaking observation of patients after cataract surgery and the development of techniques for observing the posterior vitreous and macula, including fluorescein photography, have clarified the problem greatly.

A more accurate picture of Irvine's syndrome has evolved as a result of ob-

Taken in part from Jaffe, N. S.: Cataract surgery and its complications, St. Louis, 1972, The C. V. Mosby Co.

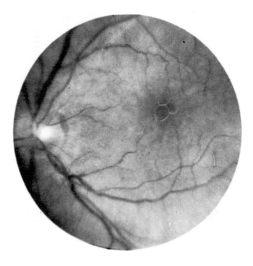

Fig. 4-1. Fundus after an uneventful lens extraction in a patient with cystoid macular edema. (From Jaffe, N. S.: The vitreous in clinical ophthalmology, St. Louis, 1969, The C. V. Mosby Co.)

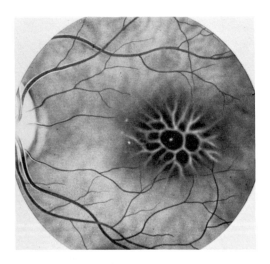

Fig. 4-2. Drawing of the fundus after an uneventful lens extraction in a patient with cystoid macular edema. (From Gass, J. D. M., and Norton, E. W. D.: Arch. Ophthalmol. **76:**646, 1966.)

servations made by Gass and Norton[8,9]: The typical patient undergoes an uneventful intracapsular cataract extraction. During the postoperative course, good visual acuity is attained; however, 1 to 3 months after surgery, visual acuity decreases to 20/50 or 20/100. The onset of this decrease may be delayed. (I have observed it more than ten years after surgery.) The eye becomes irritable and photophobic and there are recurrences and remissions of circumcorneal injection. Ophthalmoscopy (Fig. 4-1) reveals little except for loss of the foveal reflex and the presence of a yellowish reflex or spot deep in or behind the retina. The cystoid spaces are best seen by a red-free light, which renders their inner walls visible.

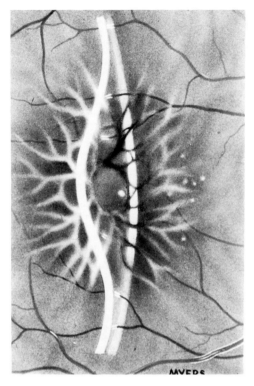

Fig. 4-3. Drawing of the biomicroscopic appearance of cystoid macular edema after a lens extraction. (From Gass, J. D. M., and Norton, E. W. D.: Arch. Ophthalmol. 76:646, 1966.)

Biomicroscopic examination with a Hruby or fundus contact lens reveals a characteristic honeycomb lesion with one or more larger cystoid spaces centrally surrounded by any number of smaller oval spaces. The glistening sections of the convex anterior walls of the cysts are seen overlying optically empty vesicles. The cysts appear to be tightly packed together, and their interfaces present a spidery pattern (Figs. 4-2 and 4-3). Small perifoveal hemorrhages are not uncommon. I have observed blood on the floor of a relatively large central cystoid space. It persisted for many months. The retina may be markedly thickened, and the lesion may occupy an area as large as one and a half or two disc diameters.

An associated serous detachment of the macula has been described,[9] but in most cases the process appears to be entirely intraretinal. A wrinkling of the inner retinal surface (pucker), resulting from contraction of a semitranslucent preretinal membrane, has been reported.[10] I have observed this several times in persisting cases of cystoid macular edema. Papilledema also may occur and be associated with peripapillary hemorrhages (Fig. 4-4).

Fluorescein angiography has proved to be of great value in diagnosing cystoid macular edema. Within 1 to 2 minutes of an antecubital vein injection of 5 ml of 10% fluorescein or 10 ml of 5% fluorescein, the dye can be observed in the

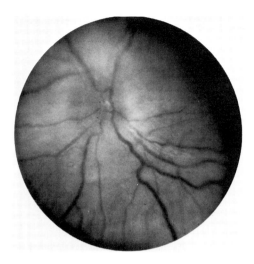

Fig. 4-4. Papilledema after a lens extraction in a patient with cystoid macular edema. (From Jaffe, N. S.: The vitreous in clinical ophthalmology, St. Louis, 1969, The C. V. Mosby Co.)

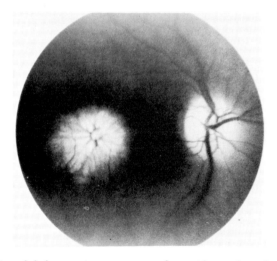

Fig. 4-5. Fluorescein ophthalmoscopic appearance of cystoid macular edema after a lens extraction. One hour after injection the central dark figure is surrounded by fluorescein pooled within intraretinal cystoid spaces. (From Gass, J. D. M., and Norton, E. W. D.: Arch. Ophthalmol. 76:646, 1966.)

macula. The macular pattern is well developed in most patients in 5 to 15 minutes although in others it requires more than 30 minutes to develop. It consists of a stellate figure with feathery margins (Fig. 4-5). The dark septa in the macular area, which compartmentalize the pattern, are probably attributable to Müller's supporting fibers of the retina. In many patients there is considerable leakage of dye into the vitreous and aqueous anteriorly, so obscuration of fundus details occurs shortly after injection; however, the pattern becomes established and

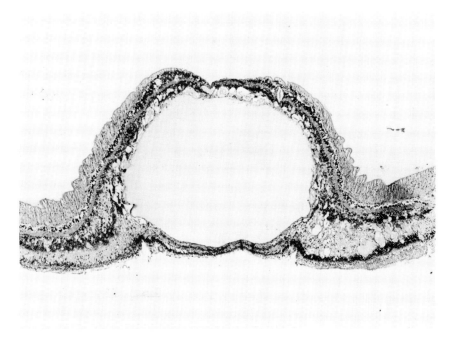

Fig. 4-6. Macular cyst after cataract extraction (×40, AFIP no. 105-3425). (From Maumenee, A. E.: Arch. Ophthalmol. **78:**151, 1967.)

visible after a short time. In patients with papilledema, there may be leakage of dye into the optic nerve and peripapillary retina. Generally, when edema of the macula and disc subsides, fluorescein leakage ceases.

An elaborate photographic setup is not available to everyone, nor is it required to make the diagnosis of cystoid macular edema. The typical fluorescein pattern may be observed with a Hruby lens or the ophthalmoscope using a no. 47 or 47A filter (Kodak Wratten). The macula will light up and become visible, even in eyes whose fundi are difficult to see because of clouding of the media.

The pathogenesis of the visual disturbance appears to involve leakage of serous exudate from intraretinal capillaries in the perifoveal area and perhaps the disc capillaries. The propensity of the macula for development of edema is based on the peculiar structure of the macula. The exudate from the incompetent capillaries forms small puddles in the outer plexiform layer of Henle, which acts like a sponge. There are usually one or more large central cystoid spaces surrounded by numerous small ones. These spaces appear to intercommunicate (Figs. 4-6 to 4-8). If papilledema is present, it is probably due to a similar leakage of serous exudate into the optic nerve head.

It may be difficult to imagine that a macula afflicted with cystoid macular edema has not lost central vision completely; yet surprisingly little visual function may actually be disturbed in the face of this ominous-appearing macula. Although permanent degenerative changes may result if the process continues unabated, most patients recover even after many months of morbidity.

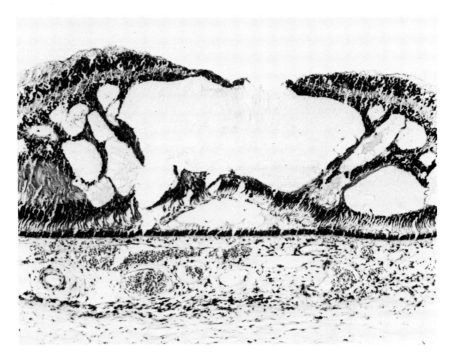

Fig. 4-7. Macular cyst after cataract extraction. The break in the inner layer of the retina is an artifact (×10, AFIP no. 119-145). (From Maumenee, A. E.: Arch. Ophthalmol. **78**:151, 1967.)

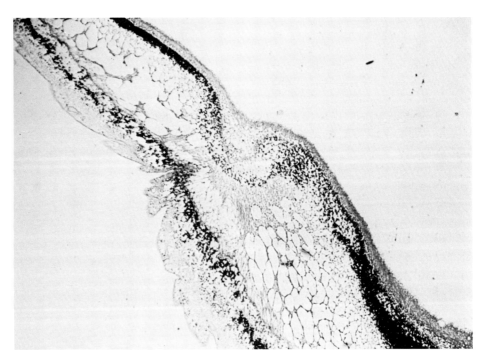

Fig. 4-8. Cystoid macular edema after cataract extraction in an eye with long-standing postoperative iridocyclitis. (From Jaffe, N. S.: Cataract surgery and its complications, St. Louis, 1972, The C. V. Mosby Co.)

The clinical appearance of the macula is not pathognomonic of the Irvine-Gass syndrome; in fact, it may occur in pars planitis, venous thrombosis, chorioretinitis, telangiectasia of the retina, and acute nongranulomatous iritis. Kolker and Becker[23] observed it after the use of topical epinephrine in aphakic patients with glaucoma. Their observation has now been confirmed. The fluorescein pattern in all these situations likewise indicates cystoid macular edema. Fluorescein leakage into the macula generally does not occur in the vitreoretinal traction syndrome or with preretinal contraction membranes—an important differential point; however, there are exceptions.

The relationship between cystoid macular edema and the occasional wrinkling of the inner retinal layer because of contraction of a semitranslucent preretinal membrane is not entirely clear. Whether the wrinkling is caused by leaking retinal vessels (as suggested by Gass and Norton[10]), whether it preexists the cataract surgery, or whether either is possible is not yet established. I have observed such membranes in patients during the early postoperative period. Since the membranes appeared to be well developed and since visual acuity at no time attained a satisfactory level, as in the Irvine-Gass syndrome, I have assumed that the maculopathy preceded the surgery.

In addition to the cystoid macular edema, there are important and significant accompanying signs: A prominent cellular infiltration in the vitreous, along with vitreous opacities, may occur—most marked posteriorly and best viewed by retroillumination. I have also noted a disruption and loss of the usual smooth contour of the posterior limiting border of the vitreous in some patients. If the term is acceptable, a *vitreitis* is the clinical picture. There is usually a circumcorneal injection, and cells are occasionally found in the aqueous. Intraocular pressure is generally normal.

In his original definition of the syndrome, Irvine[18] stated that the anterior hyaloid membrane must be ruptured; however, the same pathologic process is found in eyes with intact anterior hyaloid membranes or after an extracapsular lens extraction with an intact posterior capsule. Of sixty-four eyes with postoperative cystoid macular edema, Gass and Norton[10] observed an intact anterior hyaloid membrane in thirty-four. In thirty eyes the anterior hyaloid membrane was ruptured; and in twenty-five of these, vitreous was attached to the posterior surface of the wound.

Some authors still consider the macular lesion to be the result of vitreous traction at the posterior pole. Most recent reports[8,22,25] have discounted this since, even with the most careful technique of examination, it is extremely rare to observe vitreous fibrils attached to the cystoid lesion at the macula.

Pathogenesis

Perhaps it is too convenient to state that some patients are prone to capillary incompetence; yet Gass and Norton[10] made an interesting observation in this regard: Of forty-eight patients with postoperative cystoid macular edema thirty-two showed some evidence of existing or previous systemic hypertension.

Five of the thirty-two also had mild diabetes. Of the sixteen patients without evidence of hypertension, three had mild diabetes, one had congestive heart failure, and twelve had no history of cardiovascular disease. Thirteen of fourteen patients with persistent macular edema for one or more years had evidence of cardiovascular disease. Because of the age of the patients in this category, however, it is not known whether these observations are significant. Gass and Norton admit that a control series of patients without cystoid macular edema has not yet been studied for pertinent medical history.

It is of interest to relate these observations to the occurrence of macular edema in aphakic patients receiving topical adrenergic medication for glaucoma, as first reported by Kolker and Becker.[23] Gass and Norton[10] observed six such patients; in four the edema disappeared shortly after the medication was discontinued; and in two it disappeared spontaneously, although the medication was continued.

Apparently the etiology of cystoid macular edema remains obscure, thus inviting speculation. I have the impression that traction of the vitreous at its base may be significant. Irritability at this site may be a causative factor—in the same way that anterior segment inflammations involving the ciliary body are occasionally associated with cystoid macular edema. Biomicroscopic examination of the vitreous reveals the typical cellular infiltration, especially posteriorly. The infiltrating cells may exert a toxic influence on the relatively unprotected macula. It will be recalled that the basal lamina at the fovea is very attenuated, almost nonexistent, which could result in incompetence of the capillaries at the macula.

Equally speculative is a theory offered by Hawkins.[15] The vitreous bodies of thirty-five aphakic eyes with cystoid macular edema were studied prior to and after intravenous injection of fluorescein. Virtually all the eyes showed extensive syneresis and liquefaction of the vitreous gel and posterior detachment of the vitreous. (This is not unexpected.) Vitreomacular traction was not noted. Rupture of the anterior hyaloid membrane was present in nineteen of the thirty-five eyes. The time required for fluorescein to appear in the anterior chamber averaged 2 minutes for the involved eyes, as opposed to 10 minutes for the fellow eyes. In most cases the fluorescein then diffused into and became prominently concentrated within the collapsed vitreous gel. The findings suggested that aqueous humor proteins and electrolytes diffuse posteriorly throughout the collapsed vitreous gel. The liquefied vitreous (retrovitreal fluid) anterior to the retina assumes chemical and osmotic properties quite unlike those normally present. The result of such a change is an outpouring of fluid from the perimacular capillaries. Hawkins theorized that often after several weeks, the perimacular capillaries adjust to the osmotic imbalance and the edema clears. In eyes in which the vitreous pathology is particularly severe, however, the edema is not likely to improve. We must wonder why, if this theory is correct, myopic eyes with extensive syneresis and liquefaction of the vitreous gel do not show a higher incidence of cystoid macular edema.

Worst[37] has proposed a hypothesis attributing a number of biotoxic effects to aqueous humor. Physiologic, anatomic, and pathophysiologic observations have given him reason to assume that aqueous humor contains biochemically active principles which will manifest biotoxic effects when the aqueous leaves its natural reservoir. As a tentative name for these biotoxic principles, he has proposed the term *aqueous biotoxic complex (ABC) factors.* He attributes the lower incidence of cystoid macular edema after extracapusular lens extraction, compared to that following intracapsular extraction, to the presence of an intact posterior capsule—walling off the posterior portion of the eye from the effects of the ABC factors of the aqueous

It should be apparent from this discussion and speculation how obscure the basic pathogenesis of cystoid macular edema is at the present time.

Incidence

Irvine[18] originally reported the incidence of cystoid macular edema to be around 2%. The incidence is probably considerably higher, however, especially if searched for by the almost daily performance of visual acuity readings and frequent fundus and fluorescein evaluations.

In some patients a transient cystoid macular edema occurs but causes little disturbance since the patient has not yet been given his aphakic correction. The process may subside in a few days. It probably occurs in at least 40% of normal cataract extractions; and if it is present in one eye, there is a 70% chance it will occur in the second eye after lens extraction. In fact, if fluorescein angiography were performed daily, I would not be surprised even to find some transient phase of cystoid macular edema after every cataract extraction.

Gass and Norton[10] followed forty-eight patients for at least one year after they developed macular edema. Forty-four of them were followed for two years or longer. Of these, thirty-three had bilateral cataract extractions. Macular edema occurred in both eyes of sixteen patients, and unilaterally in seventeen.

Although the role of vitreous traction at the macula is highly doubtful, the vitreous is implicated in cystoid macular edema when any of the following occur:

1. Vitreous is lost at surgery.
2. There is a postoperative rupture of the anterior hyaloid membrane.
3. Vitreous adheres to the operative wound, especially when there is peaking of the pupil.

Cystoid macular edema is rarely encountered after glaucoma and retinal detachment surgery in which the lens is not removed and the vitreous cavity is minimally altered.

Ryan,[29] however, has described two cases of cystoid macular edema in phakic eyes after prophylactic procedures for treatment of retinal holes. In one patient the edema persisted. He also quoted Maumenee as having seen cystoid macular edema in phakic eyes after antiglaucoma filtering procedures. He suggested that this may have caused a small residual central visual field to be "snuffed out" after surgery.

In addition, there appears to be a high incidence of cystoid macular edema in aphakic eyes undergoing penetrating keratoplasty for corneal edema. Although the vitreous is frequently manipulated during this type of surgery, West and co-workers[34] found that eight of forty-two aphakic eyes with clear corneal grafts and cystoid macular edema had no vitreous manipulation during the surgery and no vitreous in the wound after the surgery.

Finally, there appears to be a low incidence of this disorder among Negroes which is difficult to explain.

Prognosis

The prognosis for full restoration of visual acuity is generally good. In most instances the macular edema is transient, with vision recovering rapidly as the process subsides; however, in a significant number of patients, the morbidity persists for a much longer period. The macula in a persistent case may seem to be so severely involved that full recovery cannot possibly occur; yet surprisingly, most of these patients do recover.

In the series reported by Gass and Norton[10] resolution of macular edema occurred within the first 6 months in about half the cases. In 20% one to three years passed before resolution, and in the remaining 30% macular edema persisted. They suggested that their findings are not an accurate reflection, however, since the incidence of intractable macular edema is probably much lower. Patients with persistent edema are more likely to be referred for consultation and are followed more closely for longer periods of time.

Jacobson and Dellaporta[20] followed twenty-eight eyes in twenty-six patients with cystoid macular edema after cataract extraction. The diagnosis was confirmed in all eyes by fluorescein angiography. Twenty-four eyes attained 20/30 or better visual acuity immediately after cataract extraction. Approximately 50% of these retained this vision for 6 months or more after surgery before it began to decrease. Twenty of the twenty-eight eyes (71.4%) had a spontaneous resolution of the cystoid macular edema and achieved 20/30 or better vision. Seven of these required 6 months or longer to clear. Eight of the twenty-eight eyes (28.6%) had 20/40 visual acuity or less. The patients were observed for two years or longer.

In the great majority of cases, the macula regains a normal appearance after subsidence of the edema; however, instances of permanent macular degeneration do arise as a consequence of prolonged persistent macular edema. Gass and Norton[10] observed two patients who developed either lamellar or full-thickness macular holes after persistent macular edema. In the absence of an operculum and of evidence of serous detachment, they assumed that a rupture in the inner retinal wall had occurred secondary to the intractable edema.

As mentioned, the cystoid spaces at the macula may coalesce so that all retinal elements, except the internal limiting membrane, disappear. When this membrane disintegrates, a lamellar hole is formed. Such a hole may measure one fourth to one third disc diameter, corresponding roughly to the size of the central avascular area. In the presence of a lamellar hole, visual acuity may be surprisingly good because of retention of some percipient elements. Occasionally it is difficult or impossible to determine biomicroscopically whether the inner layer of an apparent large foveal cystoid space is intact. Fluorescein angiography may be helpful in this situation. If the layer is intact, the stellate figure with feathery margins, as described previously, will become apparent. If a dehiscence exists, the dye will diffuse out into the vitreous cavity and the sharply circumscribed area where there is a defect in the retina will appear relatively hypofluorescent, in contrast to the surrounding fluorescent cystoid spaces (Fig. 4-9).

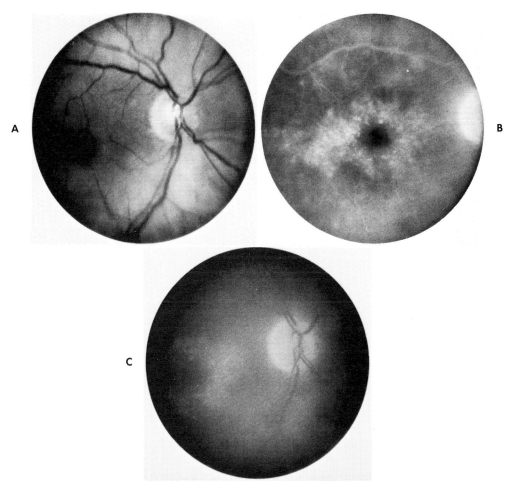

A

B

C

Fig. 4-9. **A**, Persistent macular edema and macular hole three and a half years after a cataract extraction. Visual acuity is 20/70. **B**, Intraretinal leakage of dye into the macular region. **C**, Late stage. Cystoid macular edema surrounds the central nonfluorescent area in the region of the macular hole. (From Gass, J. D. M., and Norton, E. W. D.: Trans. Am. Acad. Ophthalmol. Otolaryngol. **73**:665, 1969.)

The presence of vitreous incarceration in the wound may have some bearing on the ultimate prognosis. Gass and Norton[10] noted that patients with cystoid macular edema whose anterior hyaloid membrane remained intact recovered in an average of 6 months. Those with incarceration of vitreous in the posterior part of the wound recovered in an average 15 months. The authors reported an incidence of vitreous incarceration of 55% in patients with persistent edema and 35% in patients who recovered. My two most resistant cases were associated with operative loss of vitreous.

Treatment

As is usual with a disorder that shows a naturally high rate of recovery, a number of beneficial therapeutic remedies have been advocated. The use of systemic steroids and atropine applied topically may be of value, particularly in those cases with considerable cellular infiltration in the vitreous. In several patients I have used an injection under Tenon's capsule of triamcinolone (Kenalog) and found that it improved vision. Although their use is probably justified, to date I have not been overly impressed with triamcinolone steroids.

Tennant[31] has advocated the use of indomethacin (Indocin) in patients with cystoid macular edema. This nonsteroid anti-inflammatory compound is given orally in a dosage of 25 mg three times daily after meals. Gastrointestinal disturbances may occur in about 15% of patients taking this medication.

EDITOR'S NOTE

Dr. Lawrence A. Yannuzzi, of the Manhattan Eye, Ear & Throat Hospital, using the antiprostaglandin indomethacin or a placebo for 6 weeks in a controlled study of thirty-four patients, found no beneficial effects from the drug (personal communication, 1976).

In patients who show vitreous adherence to the surgical wound, especially with peaking of the pupil, separation of these adhesions may be of value. Iliff[17] has recommended incision of the adhesions by means of exteriorizing them with a bent 30-gauge cannula, which is inserted into the anterior chamber through a limbal stab wound so that one can cut them with scissors. Some success with this procedure has been reported. Too often, on biomicroscopic examination 1 or 2 days later, vitreous is found to have readhered to the wound at the original site or to the region of the stab wound.

In some patients solid vitreous may nearly fill the entire anterior chamber, with widespread adherence to the wound. The procedure of Iliff cannot be used on these eyes. If the cystoid macular edema has persisted for a long time and visual acuity has dropped to 20/200 or less, an alternative procedure may be attempted. The wound is reopened to the extent of a cataract incision. The vitreous is removed from the anterior chamber with a cellulose sponge (Fig. 4-10). The sponge is effective in engaging solid vitreous in the angle, over the anterior surface of the iris, and in the pupillary aperture. Large bundles of vitreous are picked up and cut (at the pupillary plane) with scissors. When sufficient vitreous has been removed, the iris will fall well posteriorly. The wound

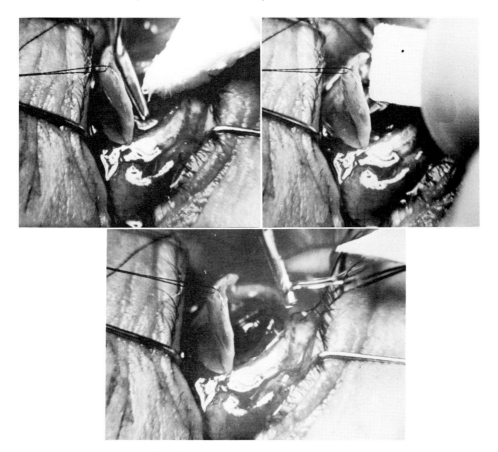

Fig. 4-10. Vitrectomy performed in a patient with cystoid macular edema associated with widespread adherence of vitreous to the wound after lens extraction. Vitreous is picked up with a cellulose sponge and cut with scissors. (From Jaffe, N. S.: The vitreous in clinical ophthalmology, St. Louis, 1969, The C. V. Mosby Co.)

is then sutured in the usual manner. The eye tolerates this procedure surprisingly well. As a rule recondensation of the face of the remaining vitreous will occur at about the level of the iris.

This method of partial anterior vitrectomy is similar to that described for the management of vitreous loss during cataract surgery and in association with a penetrating keratoplasty for treatment of aphakic bullous keratopathy caused by vitreocorneal adherence. The technique will likely be replaced by the closed system type of partial anterior vitrectomy via the pars plana, using the VISC (vitreous infusion suction cutter) or the Roto-Extractor.

Jacobson and Dellaporta,[20] in their series of twenty-eight eyes in twenty-six patients with cystoid macular edema after cataract extraction, concluded that no medical or surgical treatment has been demonstrated to improve the rate of natural spontaneous resolution of cystoid macular edema after cataract extraction.

There exists today a pronounced trend to intervene surgically when vitreous incarceration is associated with cystoid macular edema. The results achieved must be weighed against the decided tendency for spontaneous resolution of macular edema, even after prolonged periods. At this time, I have not been impressed with the results of vitreous surgery in late cases. Whether early intervention will prove effective in preventing intractable cases is not yet known. I must reemphasize that vitreous surgery appears to be a drastic procedure for a disorder that shows a high rate of spontaneous recovery. It should probably be reserved for cases persisting more than a year.

VITREORETINAL TRACTION SYNDROME

After lens extraction, alterations at the posterior pole of the fundus associated with vitreous adherent to the macula or disc are occasionally seen. Irvine[18] in 1953 ascribed the edema seen at the macula after cataract extraction to such a mechanism. This was restated more recently[32]; however, as a result of other observations,[8,22,25] it is quite conclusive that these are different entities.

In my experience vitreoretinal traction at the posterior pole of the fundus is seen far more frequently in phakic eyes—because by the time patients come to cataract surgery, they are of an age that their eyes have usually undergone a posterior vitreous detachment. Whether alterations in the vitreous associated with the cataract surgery are responsible for the vitreoretinal traction at the macula is not known. Theoretically surgery-related alterations can occur, although I have the impression that when they are encountered after cataract surgery they usually predated the surgery.

Although the relationship of the vitreoretinal traction syndrome to cataract surgery remains unclear, the presence of the traction represents another cause of failure to achieve anticipated vision as a result of alterations at the posterior pole of the fundus.

It is not surprising that the relationship of the vitreous to the posterior pole has only recently become more clearly understood, at least on a clinical basis. The availability of more sophisticated means of examining the posterior vitreous and fundus with the slit lamp has enabled the clinician to recognize these relationships. Whereas I reported fourteen patients[22] and Maumenee[25] reported seven patients with a macular pathologic condition resulting from the vitreoretinal traction syndrome, Goldmann[13] in 1958 stated that he had seen only one such case.

I repeat that if posterior pole alterations caused by vitreous traction are encountered after cataract surgery they are probably not related to the surgery itself. Nonetheless, we must recognize and understand these changes so they can be differentiated from other conditions which lend themselves to treatment and thereby obtain a clearer picture of the ultimate prognosis.

Pathogenesis

The cause of vitreoretinal adherence at the posterior pole is not known. Probably in the future a great deal more will be known about this condition and we will consider these traction phenomena to be secondary vitreoretinal adherences.

In some patients the condition may be caused by an unusually firm adherence of the vitreous to the macula. That the macula may be the site of such an adherence was noted by Grignolo,[14] who described a strong anatomic adhesion between the vitreous body and retina in the macular area. Schepens[30] stated that in the region of the disc and of the macula, separating the vitreous from the retina without breaking the surface layer or hyaloid membrane is difficult or impossible.

The exact anatomic nature of the vitreomacular relationship is still unknown although conclusions can be drawn from related histologic and clinical findings. The internal limiting membrane of the retina is not present over the nerve head but ends at the optic disc. After a posterior vitreous detachment, a prepapillary ring is present in almost every case (Fig. 4-11). It is varied in shape, but in most instances a window exists where the posterior border of the vitreous appears absent. Presumably this window, or peephole, as Vogt[33] called it, corresponds to the area over the disc.

Similarly in some cases of posterior vitreous detachment, a round or oval premacular hole (Fig. 4-12) is also present. The edge of this hole is not thickened and irregular as in the prepapillary hole, probably because the premacular hole is not surrounded by glial tissue. The internal limiting membrane is somewhat attenuated over the macula—as substantiated by Yamada's[38] electron microscopic observations that the basement membrane of the retina is approximately 1.5 μm thick at the periphery of the macula, 0.4 μm thick at the edge of the fovea, and extremely thin (10 to 15 nm) at the foveal center. The outermost vitreous fibrils are attached to the basement membrane. A possible conclusion is that the vitreous is adherent to the macula around the macular periphery but may not

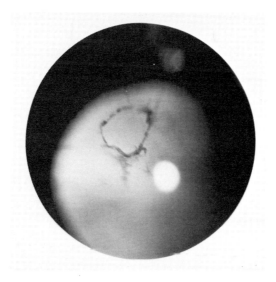

Fig. 4-11. Prepapillary opacity in a posterior vitreous detachment with collapse. (From Jaffe, N. S.: Arch. Ophthalmol. **78:**585, 1967.)

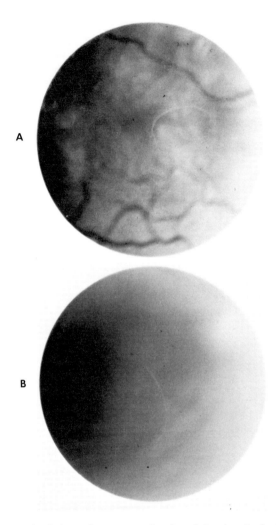

Fig. 4-12. **A,** Premacular hole in the posterior border of the detached vitreous in a 41-year-old man, representing the prior attachment of the vitreous around the macular area. **B,** Premacular hole in the posterior border of the detached vitreous in a 37-year-old woman with a posterior uveitis. (**A** from Jaffe, N. S.: Trans. Am. Acad. Ophthalmol. Otolaryngol. **71:**642, 1967; **B** from Jaffe, N. S.: Arch. Ophthalmol. **78:**585, 1967.)

have any attachment, or at best only a rudimentary attachment, to the center of the macula. The presence of a premacular hole in the posterior limiting border of the detached vitreous suggests this condition. Pathologic processes such as posterior uveitis, diabetes, and intraocular hemorrhage may cause a secondary vitreoretinal traction syndrome.

The vitreoretinal traction syndrome is more correctly a complication of posterior vitreous detachment rather than of cataract extraction. Posterior vitreous detachment may be a normal senescent process or may be associated with specific diseases (e.g., posterior uveitis, diabetes mellitus).

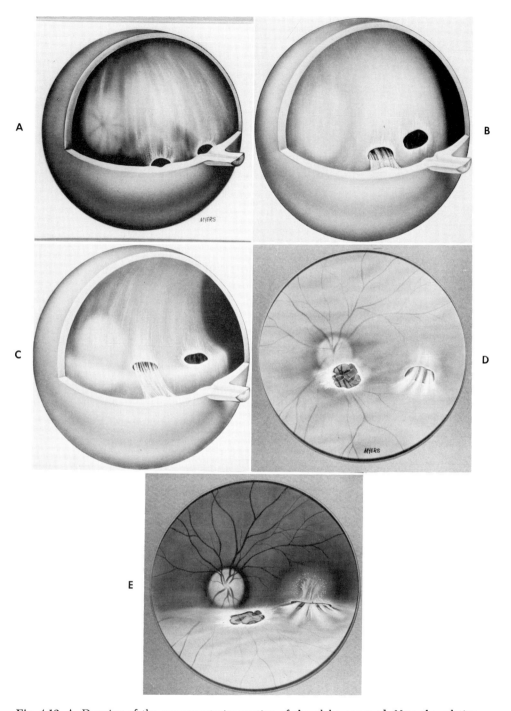

Fig. 4-13. **A,** Drawing of the superoposterior portion of the globe removed. Note the relationship of the vitreous to the disc and macula. **B** and **C,** Posterior vitreous detachment with adherence of vitreous to the macula. Collapse of the vitreous has occurred in **C,** changing the inclinations of the premacular and prepapillary holes in the posterior vitreous border. **D,** Anterior view of **B. E,** Anterior view of **C.** (**A** to **C** from Jaffe, N. S.: The vitreous in clinical ophthalmology, St. Louis, 1969, The C. V. Mosby Co.; **D** and **E** from Jaffe, N. S.: Trans. Am. Acad. Ophthalmol. Otolaryngol. **71:**642, 1967.)

Diagnosis

The diagnosis of vitreoretinal traction syndrome is made at the slit lamp with a Hruby or a fundus contact lens. The outline of the posterior vitreous detachment is traced. If the vitreous is detached from the disc, a prepapillary opacity is usually found. This opacity occupies the posterior border of the detached vitreous. The residual vitreoretinal adherence is best viewed by making the angle between the light source and the observer as wide as possible. It is to be remembered that the normal vitreous strands are slightly greater than 100 Å in diameter, which is below the normal resolution of the light microscope. Thus some vitreoretinal strands will be missed. Dark adaptation is essential for the observer in identifying smaller fibrils.

Clinical findings

The vitreoretinal traction syndrome presents several signs and symptoms. The onset is abrupt; the patient complains of one or more of the following: painless blurring of vision, metamorphopsia, photopsia, angioscotomas, and micropsia.

Examination of the posterior vitreous and fundus reveals a posterior vitreous detachment with residual adherence of the vitreous to the posterior pole (Fig. 4-13). A mild cellular reaction may be present in the posterior vitreous. The macula appears under traction and may be somewhat thickened without a detachment of the sensory epithelium of the retina. Punctate and flame-shaped hemorrhages may be found in the retinal tissue (Fig. 4-14).

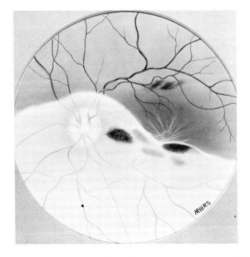

Fig. 4-14. Drawing of a posterior vitreous detachment in a 65-year-old man. There are two intraretinal hemorrhages superonasal to the macula, and five hemorrhages in the posterior border of the vitreous. Adherence of vitreous to the macula is seen. Visual acuity is 20/70. The hemorrhages disappeared in 5 days and visual acuity improved to 20/50. Three weeks later the vitreoretinal adherence separated and visual acuity was 20/30. (From Jaffe, N. S.: Arch. Ophthalmol. **78**:585, 1967.)

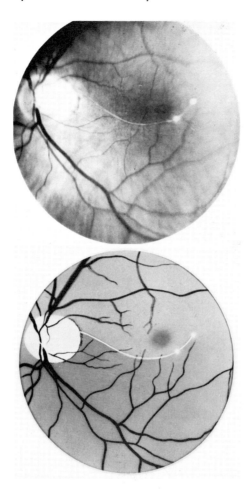

Fig. 4-15. Vitreoretinal traction syndrome. Note the horizontal line of adherence of the vitreous to the retina from the disc across the inferior portion of the macular area. The sketch emphasizes the line of adherence. (From Jaffe, N. S.: Arch. Ophthalmol. **78:**585, 1967.)

In my experience the adherence of vitreous to the posterior pole may present in one of the following four ways:

1. As a distinct horizontal line of adherence extending from the disc across the macula and out to the periphery (Fig. 4-15). The chronologic sequence of events in the pathogenesis of such a horizontal line of adherence was followed in a young adult who suffered a recurrence of a posterior uveitis (Fig. 4-16).

2. As a broad irregular adherence to the posterior pole (Fig. 4-17). The sequence of events in such a lesion and its subsequent changes are shown in Fig. 4-18.

3. As a taut strand of vitreous connecting the separated vitreous to the macula (Fig. 4-19).

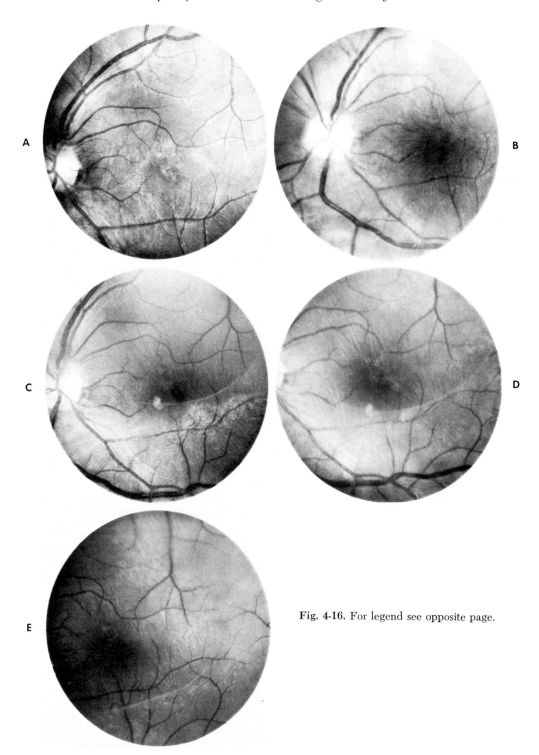

Fig. 4-16. For legend see opposite page.

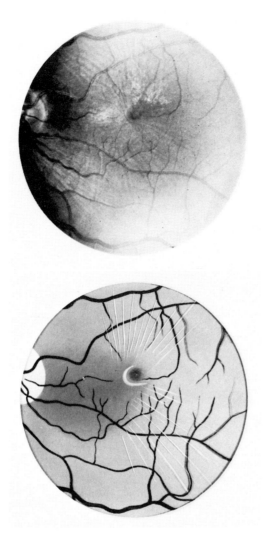

Fig. 4-17. Posterior vitreous detachment in a 40-year-old man. There is residual vitreoretinal adherence from the disc to the macula. The densest area of adherence is represented by a swirl of vitreous on the nasal and inferior margins of the fovea. Metamorphopsia is present. Visual acuity is 20/25. The sketch emphasizes the broad area of vitreous adherence and the swirl near the fovea. (From Jaffe, N. S.: Trans. Am. Acad. Ophthalmol. Otolaryngol. **71**:642, 1967.)

Fig. 4-16. Toxoplasmic chorioretinitis in a 26-year-old man. **A,** On January 7, 1966, the posterior pole of the fundus appears normal. **B,** On March 2, 1966, there are minimal traction lines nasal to the macula. Note the early separation of the vitreous superotemporally to the macula. Visual acuity is 20/20. **C,** On March 22, 1966, there is a posterior vitreous detachment with a line of vitreous adherence extending from the temporal edge of the disc across the macula and out to the periphery. Visual acuity is 20/30. **D,** On March 30, 1966, the adherent vitreous has peeled away from the macula. Visual acuity is 20/20. **E,** on April 25, 1966, the line of vitreous adherence is still more inferior. (From Jaffe, N. S.: Trans. Am. Acad. Ophthalmol. Otolaryngol. **71**:642, 1967.)

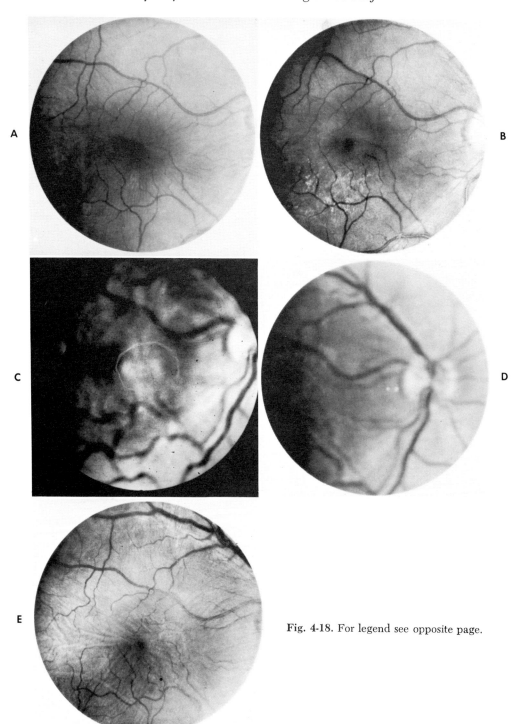

Fig. 4-18. For legend see opposite page.

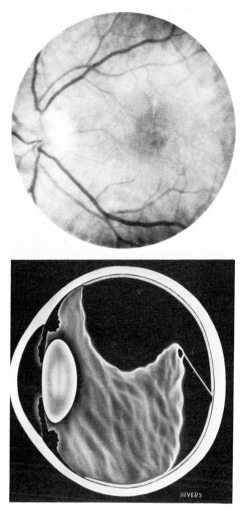

Fig. 4-19. Taut strand of vitreous attached to the macula at the edge of a macular hole in a 68-year-old man. The strand originates from the upper edge of a premacular hole in the posterior border of the detached vitreous. Visual acuity is 20/100 +2. The sketch emphasizes the residual vitreoretinal adherence. (From Jaffe, N. S.: Trans. Am. Acad. Ophthalmol. Otolaryngol. **71**:642, 1967.)

Fig. 4-18. Posterior vitreous detachment and residual vitreoretinal adherence to the paramacular area in a 41-year-old man. **A,** On October 11, 1965, visual acuity is 20/70. Metamorphopsia is present. The densest area of adherence is superonasal and inferonasal to the macula. **B,** On October 19, 1965, the adherence has separated and visual acuity has improved to 20/25 +3. Note the irregular light reflexes inferior to the macula as if the smooth contour of the inner layer of the retina has been disturbed. **C,** Premacular hole in the posterior border of the detached vitreous representing the area of prior adherence to the perimacular area. **D,** Note the prepapillary opacity in front of and slightly temporal to the disc. **E,** One year later there is marked wrinkling of the inner retina at the level of the internal limiting membrane. Visual acuity is 20/30, but the patient complains of metamorphopsia. (**A** to **C** from Jaffe, N. S.: Trans. Am. Acad. Ophthalmol. Otolaryngol. **71**:642, 1967; **D** and **E** from Jaffe, N. S.: The vitreous in clinical ophthalmology, St. Louis, 1969, The C. V. Mosby Co.)

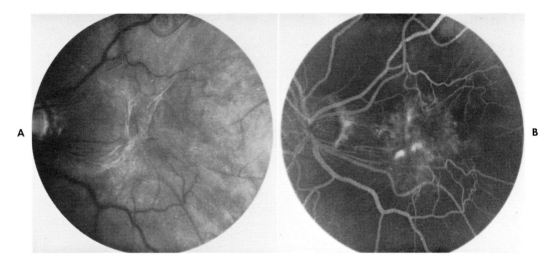

Fig. 4-20. **A,** Wrinkling of the inner layer of the retina and an extensive preretinal membrane in a 68-year-old man. Visual acuity is 20/400. **B,** Extensive leakage of dye into the macular area. (From Jaffe, N. S.: The vitreous in clinical ophthalmology, St. Louis, 1969, The C. V. Mosby Co.)

    4. As an adherence only to the disc, causing elevation with hemorrhages on or around the disc.

Fluorescein angiography usually reveals no leakage into the retinal tissue or into the subretinal space from the underlying choroid—an important point in differentiating this condition from the Irvine-Gass syndrome, serous detachment of the macula, and serous detachment of the pigment epithelium. Gass[7] observed that in patients with a greater degree of retinal wrinkling and distortion, angiography occasionally demonstrated variable degrees of intraretinal leakage of dye (Figs. 4-20 and 4-21). He noted furthermore that the pattern of dye pooling was always irregular and appeared quite different from the characteristic pattern seen in cystoid macular edema.

Prognosis

In favorable cases the vitreous peels away from the retina and the symptoms simultaneously disappear. In more intense cases, however, three important sequelae may result:

    1. Cystic degeneration of the macula

    2. A macular hole

    3. Macular pucker and preretinal membrane formation

Cystic degeneration of the macula. When vitreous adheres for a considerable period of time to the retina, a cystic degeneration may ensue (Fig. 4-22). Boniuk[1] differentiated a cystic macular edema confined mainly to the inner nuclear layer from the cystoid macular edema seen in the Irvine-Gass syndrome, which involves the outer plexiform layer of Henle. Whether this is a valid differentiation is not known at the present time.

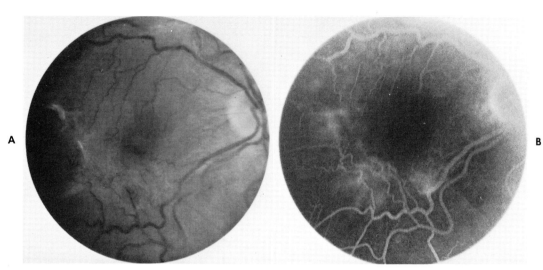

Fig. 4-21. A, Wrinkling of the inner layer of the retina and preretinal membrane formation in a 66-year-old woman. Visual acuity is 20/70. B, Extensive leakage of dye into the area of the wrinkling. (From Jaffe, N. S.: The vitreous in clinical ophthalmology, St. Louis, 1969, The C. V. Mosby Co.)

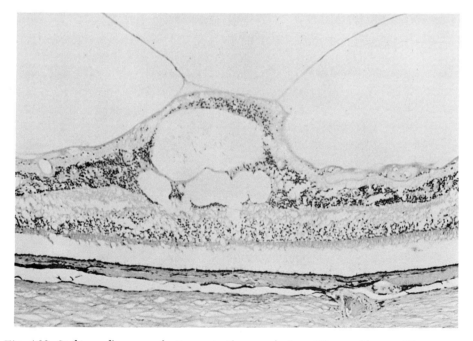

Fig. 4-22. Striking adherence of vitreous to the macula in a 75-year-old man. The eye was phakic. Cystic macular edema was confined mainly to the inner nuclear layer. (From Boniuk, M.: Survey Ophthalmol. **13**:118, 1968.)

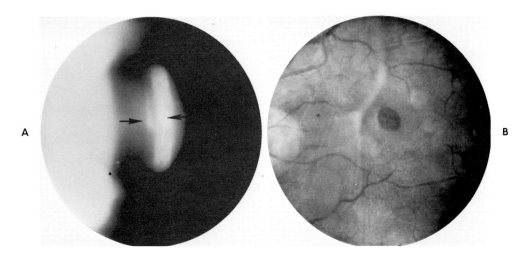

Fig. 4-23. **A,** Slit lamp photograph through a Hruby lens demonstrating vitreous (left arrow) adherent to the nasal edge of a macular hole (right arrow) in the left eye of a 74-year-old man. **B,** A band of vitreous one disc diameter nasal to the macular hole with an extension to the nasal edge of the hole. (From Jaffe, N. S.: Cataract surgery and its complications, St. Louis, 1972, The C. V. Mosby Co.)

Macular hole. Vitreomacular traction may cause a macular hole. I do not consider it a frequent cause; but when an operculum has been torn free from the macula and is adherent to a band of vitreous or when vitreous strands bridge or attach to the edge of a macular hole (Fig. 4-23), the evidence is compelling to consider this traction as a probable cause of macular hole formation.

Macular pucker and preretinal membrane formation. After the vitreous separates from the posterior pole, the symptoms usually disappear and the fundus appearance may return to normal. The examiner may be surprised at a later date, however, to observe a wrinkling of the inner layer of the retina associated with a preretinal membrane of variable thickness. The sequence of events in such a case is well exemplified in Fig. 4-18. The cause of the wrinkling and the preretinal membrane is still unknown. They may be related to the proliferation of vitreous cells in the vitreous fibrils that remain in contact with the retina after a posterior vitreous detachment.

PERSISTENT CORNEAL EDEMA SECONDARY
TO VITREOCORNEAL ADHERENCE

Persistent corneal edema from vitreocorneal adherence may occur after an uneventful lens extraction (Fig. 4-24). Its incidence is higher if cornea guttata or endothelial dystrophy exists, since vitreous (intact anterior hyaloid membrane or loose vitreous fibrils) adheres easily to damaged endothelium. The condition is particularly frustrating for both the patient and the surgeon since it may follow a well-performed operation.

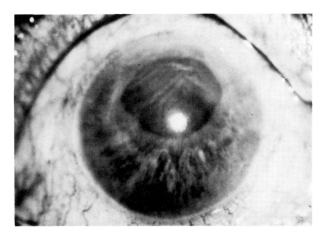

Fig. 4-24. Corneal edema after cataract extraction attributable to vitreocorneal adherence. (From Jaffe, N. S.: Cataract surgery and its complications, St. Louis, 1972, The C. V. Mosby Co.)

Emphasis cannot be too strongly placed on the key to successful management of this complication: it is early recognition. The treatment gets more complex and the prognosis worse, the longer the pathologic state exists.

In my experience this condition is usually an early complication of cataract surgery occurring in the first few postoperative days when the corneal endothelium is still suffering from surgical trauma and the bulge of the anterior hyaloid membrane is greatest. I have, however, seen several late cases occurring one or more years after cataract surgery. In these a rupture of the anterior hyaloid membrane occurred some time after surgery, and loose vitreous fibrils adhered to the back of the cornea. The cornea remained clear for a long time despite the adherence, but finally corneal edema ensued. As just described, sufficient endothelial cell damage results from the vitreous adhesion and decompensation ensues.

Pathogenesis

The causes of persistent corneal edema are varied. Chandler[2] emphasized the role of pupillary block. Either associated with or independent of pupillary block is the occurrence of an early or late flat anterior chamber. In fact, Goar[12] reported this complication in twelve of 300 intracapsular lens extractions. Eight had a late flat chamber, averaging 18 days after surgery. The condition of the corneal endothelium is also important. Damage to the corneal endothelium as a result of surgical trauma establishes a favorable environment for vitreocorneal adherence; however, the presence of corneal endothelial disease (endothelial dystrophy) prior to surgery likewise favors such an adherence. There are also a number of other factors difficult to assess.

Factors that create a bulge of the anterior hyaloid membrane must be considered (e.g., pooling of retrovitreal aqueous). I also have the impression that after chemical or mechanical zonulysis, the vitreous loses some of its support at the vitreous base. I do not believe that the vitreous ever detaches from its base; but the vitreous in this area possibly gains some freedom so that it compresses its central core, thereby creating a bulge. Paufique and Royer[27] suggested these patients may demonstrate a genetic fragility—a tempting thought which might explain bilateral cases. There appears to be a relatively high incidence of bilaterality with this complication.

Prognosis

When postoperative vitreocorneal adherence occurs I have found several prognostic factors useful. It is helpful to clear the cornea with topically administered glycerin to obtain a proper estimate of the vitreocorneal relationship at the slit lamp.

The following acronym helps in remembering these prognostic factors:

L-A-D-D-E

1. **Location of the contact.** Generally adherence of vitreous to the center of the cornea is far more serious than adherence to the periphery of the cornea (Figs. 3-1 and 3-2).
2. **Area of the contact.** Generally the greater the area of adherence, the poorer will be the prognosis. The area of contact frequently appears larger than it really is. The actual portions of the adherence are usually marked by lines of adherence oriented horizontally or obliquely—like elevated ridges, as if the vitreous is tugging at the back of the cornea. The remainder of the area of contact is mere apposition and not true adherence. This may be demonstrated by having the patient look up and down. The vitreous will roll on and off the cornea with these movements.
3. **Duration of the contact.** The longer the persistence of the vitreocorneal adherence, the poorer is the prognosis.
4. **Density of the contact.** Density is estimated by the ease with which mydriatics and systemically administered hyperosmotic agents effect a separation of the adherence.
5. **Endothelium.** The status of the corneal endothelium is probably the most important prognostic factor. Included is preoperative corneal disease (endothelial dystrophy) as well as postoperative corneal alterations caused by surgical trauma. Clinical experience tells us that loose vitreous fibrils in contact with a normal cornea, after postoperative rupture of the anterior hyaloid membrane, do not cause persistent corneal edema whereas, if the endothelium is diseased or damaged, this complication does result. Many exceptions exist, however. Loose vitreous fibrils may cause this complication in one patient but not in another due to individual variations in endothelial cell concentration, as discussed previously. Materials such as blood, vitreous, lint, rubber, and suture material adhere with great ease to the dystrophic cornea.

It is a pity that we possess no reliable means of predicting which corneas with guttatae will proceed to develop endothelial dystrophy of the Fuchs type.

Clinical course

The course of this problem is a relentless progression of corneal edema, bullous keratopathy, and late opacification. As described previously, when vitreous adheres to the cornea for a considerable period of time, the endothelial cells enlarge and eventually disappear—thus depriving the cornea of its pump mechanism. Stromal edema occurs and causes positive stromal fluid pressure, which favors epithelial edema. Apparently, therefore, these cases must be discovered early since late treatment is usually ineffective in reversing the corneal edema,

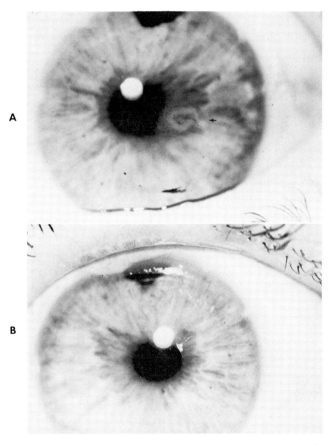

Fig. 4-25. Corneal dystrophy (Fuchs'). **A,** Left eye after an intracapsular lens extraction. There was vitreocorneal adherence just temporal to the pupil (arrow). This localized area of bullous keratopathy persisted for five years without spreading across the cornea. No postoperative oral glycerin was used. Visual acuity is 20/30. **B,** Right eye after an intracapsular lens extraction. Oral glycerin was administered postoperatively for 4 days. There was no vitreocorneal adherence. Visual acuity is 20/30. (From Jaffe, N. S.: The vitreous in clinical ophthalmology, St. Louis, 1969, The C. V. Mosby Co.)

even if the vitreocorneal adherence is terminated. As an aid to early diagnosis, glycerin is applied topically to clear the cornea; in extreme cases the corneal epithelium may be denuded.

Treatment
Prophylactic

Various prophylactic measures are available for patients in whom the first eye suffers persistent corneal edema or when an early preoperative corneal dystrophy exists (Fig. 4-25).

Medical

When vitreocorneal adherence is detected early, medical therapy may be effective. I have occasionally been successful in terminating the adherence by administering a hyperosmotic agent (glycerin orally or mannitol intravenously).[21] These agents effect a posterior displacement of the anterior hyaloid membrane, presumably by a reduction of vitreous volume. Mydriatics are used in conjunction to minimize pupillary block.

Surgical

Modified Leahey procedure. The best treatment in an early case is that recommended by Leahey[24] (Figs. 4-26 and 4-27). I prefer to use a 25-gauge Rizzuti-Spirizzi cannula needle attached to a syringe to perforate the sclera through the pars plana, 5 mm from the limbus. While I aspirate on the syringe, the needle enters the vitreous in its posterosuperior portion. When the needle penetrates the posterior limiting border of the vitreous, a gush of retrovitreal fluid enters the syringe. About 1 or 2 ml are withdrawn. The needle is then removed, and the pars planotomy site does not have to be sutured. The need for a sharp needle is emphasized in Fig. 4-28.

Air is then forced into the anterior chamber by the same cannula needle, which enters the anterior chamber through the limbus in the inferior temporal quadrant. If the bubble of air is fragmented by residual strands of adherent vitreous, the adhesion may have to be broken with an iris spatula introduced through the enlarged limbal wound. I have found that this is rarely necessary. If pupillary block is present, a peripheral iridectomy or anterior vitrotomy may be performed through the incision. When the air has successfully separated the vitreous from the cornea, acetylcholine is introduced into the anterior chamber and the large air bubble is left in place.

The miosis is of benefit since it lessens the chances of a readherence of vitreous to the cornea and of an air block glaucoma due to air getting behind the iris and into the vitreous. The limbal wound is closed with a single suture. Postoperatively glycerin is administered orally every 12 hours for 4 days and mydriatics are prescribed.

This surgical approach is effective in early cases (Fig. 4-29) and in an oc-

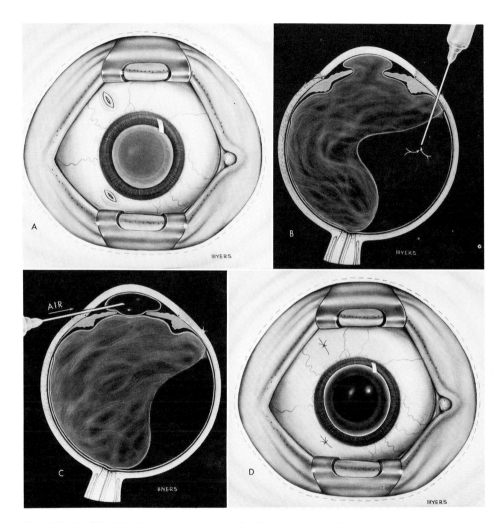

Fig. 4-26. Modified Leahey procedure. **A,** Scleral groove 2 mm from the limbus in the inferior temporal quadrant. **B,** Fluid is aspirated from the retrovitreal space via a pars planotomy through the upper scleral incision. An 18-gauge needle is used. **C,** Air is pushed into the anterior chamber after the lower scleral incision is completed into the anterior chamber as in a cyclodialysis. **D,** Completion of the procedure with air in the anterior chamber and scleral incisions sutured. (From Jaffe, N. S.: The vitreous in clinical ophthalmology, St. Louis, 1969, The C. V. Mosby Co.)

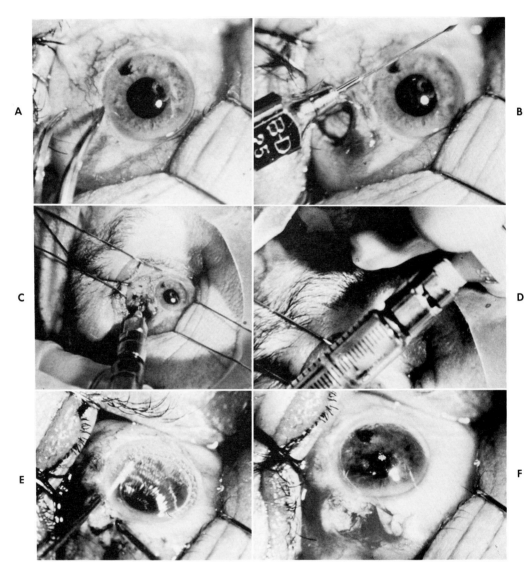

Fig. 4-27. Modified Leahey procedure for early treatment of corneal edema from vitreocorneal adherence. **A,** Mark made 5 mm from the limbus in the superotemporal quadrant at the site of the posterior sclerotomy. **B,** Rizzuti-Spirizzi 25-gauge cannula needle. **C,** Aspiration of fluid vitreous from the retrovitreal space. **D,** Air from the operating room sterilized by collecting through a Millipore filter. **E,** Air injected into the anterior chamber through the limbal wound. **F,** Miosis achieved after irrigation of acetylcholine solution into the anterior chamber. The anterior chamber remains filled with air. (From Jaffe, N. S.: Cataract surgery and its complications, St. Louis, 1972, The C. V. Mosby Co.)

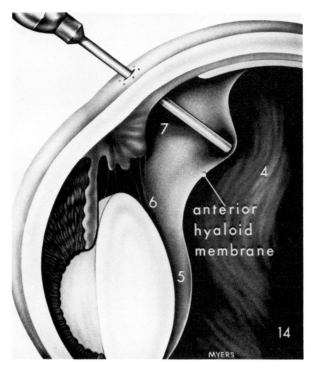

Fig. 4-28. Demonstration of the need for a sharp-tipped rather than a blunt-tipped needle in aspirating fluid from the retrovitreal space. *4,* Formed vitreous; *5,* Berger's space; *6,* canal of Petit; *7,* hyaloideo-orbicular space (Garnier); *14,* retrovitreal space. (Modified from Cibis, P. A.: Vitreoretinal pathology and surgery in retinal detachment, St. Louis, 1965, The C. V. Mosby Co.)

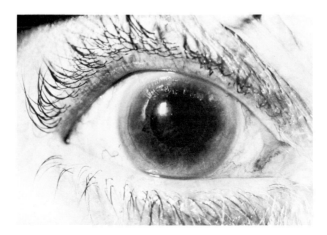

Fig. 4-29. Ideal circumstance for the Leahey treatment. Eye 2 weeks after an intracapsular lens extraction complicated by corneal edema and bullous keratopathy due to vitreocorneal adherence. (From Jaffe, N. S.: The vitreous in clinical ophthalmology, St. Louis, 1969, The C. V. Mosby Co.)

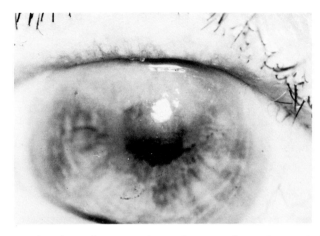

Fig. 4-30. One year after the performance of a Leahey procedure. This eye had previously undergone an intracapsular lens extraction complicated by persistent corneal edema, bullous keratopathy, and almost total corneal opacification. Visual acuity was 10/400. The Leahey procedure was performed 4 months after the lens extraction. The lower half of the cornea cleared, and visual acuity improved to 20/40. (From Jaffe, N. S.: The vitreous in clinical ophthalmology, St. Louis, 1969, The C. V. Mosby Co.)

casional late case (Fig. 4-30). After 3 to 4 weeks, however the chances for a surgical success fall sharply.

Partial anterior vitrectomy via the pars plana. A new and effective method of removing vitreous from the anterior chamber without opening the original cataract wound is via a pars plana approach. The instrument of either Dr. Machemer (VISC—vitreous infusion suction cutter) or Dr. Douvas (Roto-Extractor) promises to replace the Leahey procedure since it can safely rid the back of the cornea of adherent vitreous through a relatively small pars plana incision. At the present time I am aware of several successful applications of this method for such a complication. The technique will not likely suffer the fate of many promising modalities since it has had several years of successful trials in the posterior vitreous for removal of opaque material (e.g., organized hemorrhage, amyloid) and for removing traction bands in retinal detachment.

Cryotherapy. Drysdale and Shea[3] recommended the use of a cryoapplicator applied to the cornea. The cryoapplicator destroys the endothelium, permitting the vitreous to retract. Regeneration of the corneal endothelium occurs, resulting in a cure. If pupillary block is present, it is combined with an iridectomy. The authors reported success in a single case. I have had no experience with this technique; but I would urge extreme caution, since a permanent and total corneal decompensation may result. This technique has not gained much popularity in the ten years following its introduction.

Partial anterior vitrectomy via the open sky technique. I have occasionally seen patients who developed corneal edema one or more years after cataract extraction and in whom there occurred, soon after surgery, a rupture of the anterior hyaloid membrane with adherence of loose vitreous strands to the back of the cornea. These eyes fare well for some time but then develop intermittent bouts of corneal edema. Close inspection reveals that the vitreous conglomerates in the anterior chamber have thickened and their adhesions on the back of the cornea have become more apparent.

Typically the occurrences of corneal edema become more frequent and more prolonged, for the reasons discussed earlier. In these late cases I have found the Leahey procedure to be useless. I have occasionally been successful in terminating the edema by performing an anterior vitrectomy. If the endothelial cell population is markedly attenuated, however, this procedure will be ineffective.

In performing the open sky technique, a 180° section is made. The cornea is retracted with a retraction suture. A cellulose sponge engages bundles of formed vitreous, which are excised. As the vitreous is drawn out of the anterior chamber, strands peel off the back of the cornea. Vitreous is removed from the surface of the iris and from the pupillary area until the anterior surface of the remaining vitreous assumes a concave shape behind the level of the iris and the iris drops back. A considerable amount of vitreous may be removed by this procedure. It is surprising how well the eye tolerates the manipulation. Postoperatively the anterior surface of the vitreous recondenses but usually does not readhere to the cornea.

In two patients, respectively, the edema recurred 5 weeks and 4 months postoperatively. In two others the corneas have remained clear more than one year after the surgery. This technique will likely be replaced by partial anterior vitrectomy through the pars plana approach.

Penetrating keratoplasty. In late cases of persistent corneal edema, a penetrating keratoplasty offers the best hope for visual rehabilitation. Twenty years ago persistent corneal edema would have been considered an unfavorable condition for keratoplasty. There still may be no unanimity among ophthalmologists and even among keratoplasty surgeons that bullous keratopathy associated with vitreocorneal adherence is favorably managed by a corneal transplantation. My personal experience and the experiences of colleagues with whom I carry on a continuous dialogue on this subject are that 70% or more of these cases may be successfully grafted.

I have the impression that the improved prognosis is attributable to (1) more satisfactory suture material, (2) better instrumentation, and (3) improved methods of preventing readherence of vitreous to the cornea. In estimating prognosis, however, one must bear in mind that these cases may be complicated by more than vitreous adherence. There may be extensive anterior iris adhesions (Fig. 4-31), corneal vascularization (Fig. 4-32), and glaucoma. Anterior iris adhesions may be managed at surgery unless they are very extensive. Corneal vascularization offers less hope for successful treatment. If glaucoma is present, the outlook is gloomy.

Another impression I have is that such grafts show a tendency to late clouding. In these instances the recurrence of corneal edema is not usually associated

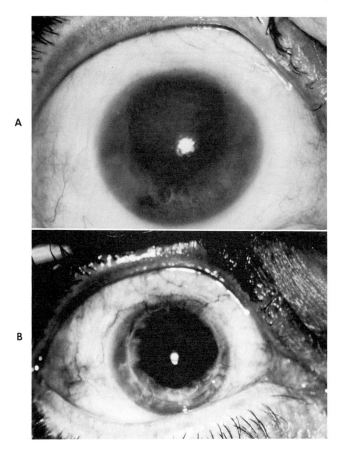

Fig. 4-31. A, Marked corneal edema after an intracapsular lens extraction complicated by vitreocorneal adherence. Iris is adherent to the cornea at 7 o'clock. B, After an 8 mm penetrating keratoplasty with removal of all vitreous from the anterior chamber. The corneal graft remains clear. (From Jaffe, N. S.: The vitreous in clinical ophthalmology, St. Louis, 1969, The C. V. Mosby Co.)

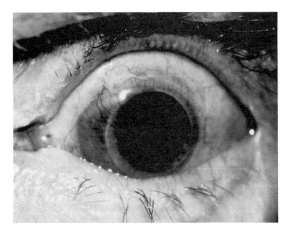

Fig. 4-32. A 7 mm penetrating keratoplasty was performed for corneal edema, bullous keratopathy, extensive adhesions of iris to the cornea, and widespread corneal vascularization after an intracapsular lens extraction. The corneal graft remains clear. (From Jaffe, N. S.: The vitreous in clinical ophthalmology, St. Louis, 1969, The C. V. Mosby Co.)

with a readherence of vitreous to the back of the cornea. Although I am unaware of a reported series of cases, some eyes that have been successfully grafted have developed problems after three to five years. This impression, however, must be tempered by the fact that most of these patients were elderly and a few years of good vision was very meaningful. Many late failures, in addition, have been successfully regrafted.

For as yet unexplained reasons, there appears to be a relatively high incidence of cystoid macular edema after aphakic keratoplasty. This was emphasized in a report[34] stating that of forty-two eyes, fourteen had a combined cataract extraction and penetrating keratoplasty and twenty-eight had a penetrating keratoplasty some time after the cataract extraction. Twenty-seven of the forty-two eyes (64%) developed cystoid macular edema. The authors stressed that eight eyes which had had no vitreous manipulation during surgery or postoperative vitreous in the wound developed cystoid macular edema or a diffuse macular edema. I have also been aware of a relatively high incidence of cystoid macular edema in such patients. When the graft remains clear, however, the patient is usually pleased with his vision since the preoperative visual acuity is generally between 20/800 and hand motion and the postoperative acuity between 20/30 and 20/60 in spite of the presence of cystoid macular edema.

I have experienced the opposite situation at least twice. In two patients with aphakic bullous keratopathy and angiographically proved cystoid macular edema, there was no cystoid macular edema after penetrating keratoplasty and partial anterior vitrectomy. One of these cases is worthy of discussion. A 71-year-old man had phthisis bulbi in one eye following an expulsive hemorrhage several days after cataract extraction. The second eye had a cataract extraction which was complicated by persistent corneal edema, probably due to vitreocorneal adherence. When the patient was first seen 6 months after the second extraction, visual acuity had improved to 20/800 in spite of relatively good clearing of the cornea with a topically administered hyperosmotic agent. Fluorescein angiography revealed 4+ cystoid macular edema. Since the eye was not painful, a keratoplasty was decided against on the basis that it would not improve vision sufficiently to warrant the risk of surgery on this patient's only eye. Within three years the cornea opacified and painful bullous keratopathy ensued. A bandage soft contact lens was fitted for continuous wear. There was no improvement in vision and the cornea was invaded by vessels. After the vision decreased to hand motion at 6 feet, an 8 mm penetrating keratoplasty and partial anterior vitrectomy were performed. Postoperative visual acuity improved to 20/30 and has remained at this level for more than five years. There has been no evidence of cystoid macular edema at any time during the postoperative course.

The technique I currently follow is to perform a 7 to 8 mm penetrating keratoplasty. The recipient corneal button is excised with vitreous attached to its back surface. Vitreous is removed from the anterior chamber with a cellulose sponge (as previously described). These sponges are far more effective than

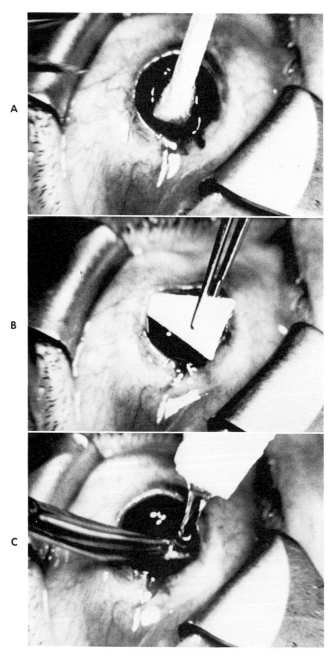

Fig. 4-33. A, Penetrating keratoplasty performed for persistent corneal edema caused by vitreo-corneal adherence after a lens extraction. The vitreous is drawn up from the anterior chamber with a cellulose sponge. **B,** Vitreous removed from the angle of the anterior chamber. **C,** Formed vitreous picked up with a cellulose sponge is excised with scissors. (From Jaffe, N. S.: The vitreous in clinical ophthalmology, St. Louis, 1969, The C. V. Mosby Co.)

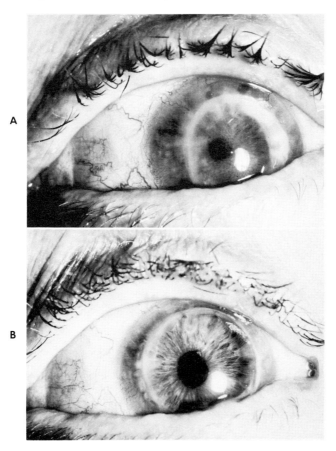

Fig. 4-34. **A,** Keratoplasty was performed for persistent corneal edema caused by vitreocorneal adherence after a lens extraction. In this case vitreous was not excised from the anterior chamber. The corneal graft became edematous. **B,** Keratoplasty was performed again. Vitreous was this time completely removed from the anterior chamber. The corneal graft remains clear. (From Jaffe, N. S.: The vitreous in clinical ophthalmology, St. Louis, 1969, The C. V. Mosby Co.)

forceps or a cryoprobe in picking up the vitreous. Formed vitreous is removed from the angle, from the surface of the iris, and from the pupillary area (Fig. 4-33). When the iris falls back posteriorly, sufficient vitreous has been removed. I usually perform two or three peripheral iridotomies. The donor button is sutured in place, preferably with the aid of an operating microscope. The surgical results have been impressive (Figs. 4-34 to 4-37).

I have achieved improved results with the following suture technique: Eight interrupted, uniformly separated, deeply inserted, edge-to-edge 10-0 nylon sutures are placed. Wide bites are taken, especially in the edematous host cornea. A continuous 10-0 nylon suture is then inserted, two bites between each interrupted suture. It is then tightened, one loop at a time, and tied at its origin. The interrupted sutures are removed in 4 to 6 weeks. The continuous suture is left in place permanently, unless the cornea surrounding it becomes vascularized.

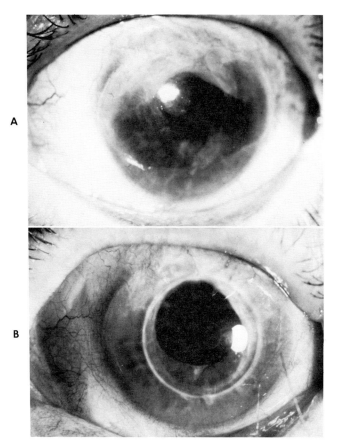

Fig. 4-35. **A,** Marked corneal edema and bullous keratopathy after an intracapsular lens extraction complicated by vitreocorneal adherence. **B,** After a 7 mm penetrating keratoplasty with removal of all vitreous from the anterior chamber. The corneal graft remains clear. (From Jaffe, N. S.: The vitreous in clinical ophthalmology, St. Louis, 1969, The C. V. Mosby Co.)

Many keratoplasty surgeons manage the vitreous differently. For example, some remove vitreous through the pars plana. I prefer the method previously outlined because I am more certain to evacuate the anterior chamber of vitreous. Condensation of the remaining vitreous usually occurs at or behind the plane of the iris. It is rare for extensive readherence of vitreous to the back of the cornea, a serious complication, to occur after an anterior vitrectomy.

It is reemphasized that early recognition of this complication after cataract surgery and early reparative surgery will usually make extensive surgical therapy unnecessary.

There are occasions when the surgeon must settle for something less than improvement in visual acuity. These are instances of painful bullous keratopathy. If the visual acuity in the opposite eye is sufficient to meet the patient's needs, he may be satisfied with only a reduction of pain. Three methods are useful toward this end:

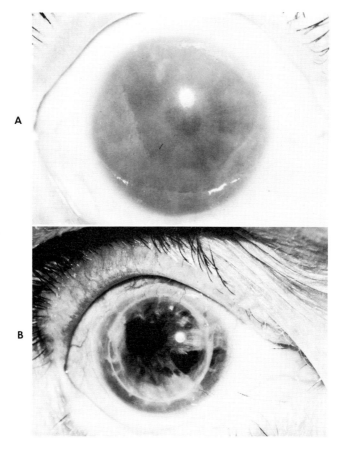

Fig. 4-36. Persistent corneal edema 11 months after an uneventful intracapsular lens extraction in a 71-year-old woman. **A,** The postoperative course was complicated by corneal edema associated with adherence of vitreous to the central area of the cornea. The iris was also adherent to the cornea at 4 o'clock. **B,** Ten months after an 8 mm penetrating keratoplasty. The portion of iris adherent to the cornea at 4 o'clock was excised, and vitreous removed from the anterior chamber. There was postoperative adherence of iris to the keratoplasty incision at 10 o'clock. (From Jaffe, N. S.: The vitreous in clinical ophthalmology, St. Louis, 1969, The C. V. Mosby Co.)

1. Hydrophilic contact lenses
2. Cautery of Bowman's membrane
3. Gundersen conjunctival flap

Hydrophilic contact lenses. Although early enthusiasts endorsed hydrophilic contact lenses for the improvement of visual acuity, I have found them disappointing in this regard in eyes with corneal edema. Unless the edema is confined to the epithelium, these lenses are usually ineffective in improving vision. Most of the eyes have corneal stromal involvement with some opacification, which is not lessened by hydrophilic lenses. The lenses frequently are effective in reducing the pain of bullous keratopathy, however.

The hydrophilic contact lenses currently available in the United States are

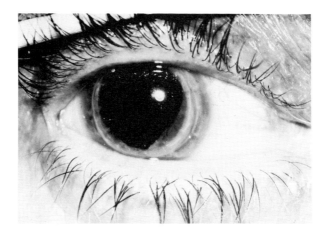

Fig. 4-37. Clear corneal graft 13 months after an 8 mm penerating keratoplasty. This 75-year-old eye had persistent corneal edema associated with vitreocorneal adherence after an intracapsular lens extraction. A portion of iris adherent to the cornea inferiorly was excised. (From Jaffe, N. S.: The vitreous in clinical ophthalmology, St. Louis, 1969, The C. V. Mosby Co.)

greatly improved over the original Czechoslovakian prototypes and are manufactured by the Warner Lambert Company. Undoubtedly newer and better lenses will become available.

The Warner Lambert bandage lens may be used in eyes which require topical medication. Hyperosmotic solutions may be applied with the lens in situ, and visual acuity may be improved to a small degree although not to the extent originally advertized.

The material used in these lenses is poly-2-hydroxyethylmethacrylate (HEMA). A polymer results when pure HEMA is polymerized in the presence of a bifunctional monomer such as ethylene glycol dimethacrylate (EGDM) to form a three-dimensional network of hydroxyethylmethacrylate chains cross-linked occasionally with diester molecules—approximately one in every 200 monomer units as an average.

The following properties make the lenses useful in ophthalmology:
1. Softness
2. Optical suitability
3. Ability to absorb water, with a concomitant swelling to a soft mass of good mechanical strength
4. Complete transparency
5. Ability to retain shape and dimensions when equilibrated in a given fluid
6. Shape recovery after deformation

Although the soft hydrophilic lenses contain water, there is no satisfactory exchange of fluid and nutrients through them. Fluid and nutrients must come by tear flow and other means. The lenses do not overcome astigmatism greater than 1.50 D. At the present time no normal eye medications can be used when these lenses (especially the Bionite lens) are worn since the lenses will absorb the medication, concentrate the preservative, and damage the corneal epithelium.[11] Thus fluorescein will permanently stain the lenses and glaucoma eyedrops are also contraindicated. This drawback, however, is somewhat compensated by the fact that hypertonic solutions can be used along with the lenses.

Not only is the anterior irregular astigmatism relieved, but the stromal swelling and haze, which can increase with an impermeable anterior surface barrier, are decreased when the soft lenses and hypertonic solutions are combined. Similarly the reduced corneal thickness with the hypertonic agents decreases the Descemet's folds and the interference of these folds with vision.[11]

For therapeutic purposes soft hydrophilic contact lenses have been comfortably and successfully worn over pathologic and irregular corneal epithelium. Their beneficial effect in these cases has been attributed to the fact that they contain almost half their own weight in water. Therefore the hydrated lens used over the dry cornea acts as a precorneal source of fluid, besides protecting the cornea against exogenous trauma and eliminating the irregular astigmatism.

The soft hydrophilic contact lenses provide the patient with bullous keratopathy rapid relief of pain. The mechanism by which the soft lenses relieve pain in bullous keratopathy is not clear, but they are of unquestionable benefit in this regard. They may be worn day and night for long periods of time. Some of the initial enthusiasm for continuous wear, however, must be tempered by the fact that a significant number of edematous corneas become dangerously vascularized. Also there have been reports of corneal ulcers developing while the lenses were in place. Nevertheless, the indications and results of the lenses will come into sharper focus in the near future.

Cautery of Bowman's membrane. A second effective method of eliminating pain in aphakic bullous keratopathy is cautery of Bowman's membrane. An excellent instructive report of this technique was provided[5] when 100 eyes with painful bullous keratopathy were treated. After scraping the corneal epithelium, the authors placed an average of 700 cautery applications to Bowman's membrane with the Bovie electrosurgical unit. The unit was set for diathermy applications and power controls set to 0. A blunt-tipped diathermy probe was used. Light and electron microscopy demonstrated an extensive subepithelial connective tissue—probably formed by an extension of the stromal connective tissue through breaks in Bowman's membrane. They suggested that the ground substance in this new tissue was responsible for an increased resistance to edema fluid and prevention of subepithelial bullae. Nearly 98% of their patients had marked to complete relief of pain.

Gundersen conjunctival flap. A thin Gundersen flap is another effective method of eliminating pain in bullous keratopathy. Although effective for symptomatic relief, this technique usually leaves the patient with ptosis of the upper eyelid.

REFERENCES

1. Boniuk, M.: Cystic macular edema secondary to vitreo-retinal traction, Survey Ophthalmol. 13:118, 1968.
2. Chandler, P. A.: Complications after

cataract extraction: clinical aspects, Trans. Am. Acad. Ophthalmol. Otolaryngol. 58:382, 1954.
3. Drysdale, I. O., and Shea, M.: Cryolysis

of adhesion of anterior hyaloid membrane to corneal endothelium after uncomplicated cataract extraction, Arch. Ophthalmol. **76**:4, 1966.

4. Duke-Elder, S.: System of ophthalmology. Vol. X, Diseases of the retina, St. Louis, 1967, The C. V. Mosby Co.

5. Farris, R. L., Iwamoto, T., and DeVoe, A. G.: Cautery of Bowman's membrane, Am. J. Ophthalmol. **77**:548, 1974.

6. Favre, M.: Trou dans la macule et décollement de la rétine, Ophthalmologica **140**:94, 1960.

7. Gass, J. D. M.: Stereoscopic atlas of macular diseases. A funduscopic and angiographic presentation, St. Louis, 1970, The C. V. Mosby Co.

8. Gass, J. D. M., and Norton, E. W. D.: Cystoid macular edema and papilledema following cataract extraction: a fluorescein funduscopic and angiographic study, Arch. Ophthalmol. **76**:646, 1966.

9. Gass, J. D. M., and Norton, E. W. D.: Fluorescein studies of patients with macular edema and papilledema following cataract extraction, Trans. Am. Ophthalmol. Soc. **64**:232, 1966.

10. Gass, J. D. M., and Norton, E. W. D.: Follow-up study of cystoid macular edema following cataract extraction, Trans. Am. Acad. Ophthalmol. Otolaryngol. **73**:665, 1969.

11. Gasset, A. R., and Kaufman, H. E.: Therapeutic uses of hydrophilic contact lenses, Am. J. Ophthalmol. **69**:252, 1970.

12. Goar, E. L.: Postoperative hyaloid adhesions to the cornea, Am. J. Ophthalmol. **45**:99, 1958.

13. Goldmann, H.: Le corps vitré. In Busacca, A., Goldmann, H., and Schiff-Wertheimer, S. P., editors: Biomicroscopie du corps vitré et du fond de l'oeil, Paris, 1957, Masson & Cie., Editeurs.

14. Grignolo, A.: Fibrous components of the vitreous body, Arch. Ophthalmol. **47**:760, 1952.

15. Hawkins, R. E.: Aphakic macular edema. In Emery, J., and Paton, D., editors: Current concepts in cataract surgery: selected proceedings of the Third Biennial Cataract Surgical Congress, St. Louis, 1974, The C. V. Mosby Co.

16. Henkind, P.: Microcirculation of the peripapillary retina, Trans. Am. Acad. Ophthalmol. Otolaryngol. **73**:890, 1969.

17. Iliff, C. E.: Treatment of the vitreous-tug syndrome, Am. J. Ophthalmol. **62**:856, 1966.

18. Irvine, S. R.: A newly defined vitreous syndrome following cataract surgery interpreted according to recent concepts of the structure of the vitreous, Am. J. Ophthalmol. **36**:599, 1953.

19. Iwanoff, A.: Beiträge zur normalen und pathologischen Anatomie des Auges. 3, Das Oedem der Netzhaut, Graefe. Arch. Ophthalmol. **15**(Abt. 2):88, 1869.

20. Jacobson, D. R., and Dellaporta, A.: Natural history of cystoid macular edema after cataract extraction, Am. J. Ophthalmol. **77**:445, 1974.

21. Jaffe, N. S., and Light, D. S.: Treatment of postoperative cataract complications by osmotic agents, Arch. Ophthalmol. **75**:370, 1966.

22. Jaffe, N. S.: Vitreous traction at the posterior pole of the fundus due to alterations in the vitreous posterior, Trans. Am. Acad. Ophthalmol. Otolaryngol. **71**:642, 1967.

23. Kolker, A. E., and Becker, B.: Epinephrine maculopathy, Arch. Ophthalmol. **79**:552, 1968.

24. Leahey, B. D.: Bullous keratitis from vitreous contact, Arch. Ophthalmol. **46**:22, 1951.

25. Maumenee, A. E.: Further advances in the study of the macula, Arch. Ophthalmol. **78**:151, 1967.

26. Michaelson, I., and Campbell, A. C. P.: The anatomy of the finer retinal vessels, and some observations on their significance in certain retinal diseases, Trans. Ophthalmol. Soc. U. K. **60**:71, 1940.

27. Paufique, L., and Royer, J.: Complications post-opératoires survenant après une extraction du cristallin et du vitré antérieur, Ann. Ocul. **193**:545, 1960.

28. Reese, A. B., Jones, I. S., and Cooper, W. C.: Macular changes secondary to vitreous traction, Trans. Am. Ophthalmol. Soc. **64**:123, 1966.

29. Ryan, S.: Cystoid maculopathy in phakic retinal detachment procedures, Am. J. Ophthalmol. **76**:519, 1973.

30. Schepens, C. L.: Clinical aspects of pathologic changes in the vitreous body, Am. J. Ophthalmol. **38**(2):8, 1954.

31. Tennant, J. L.: Personal communication, 1974.

32. Tolentino, F. I., and Schepens, C. I.: Edema of posterior pole after cataract extraction: a biomicroscopic study, Arch. Ophthalmol. **74**:781, 1965.

33. Vogt, A.: Handbook and atlas of the slit lamp microscopy of the living eye. Translation of vol. 3, ed. 2, Atlas of slit lamp microscopy, Zurich, 1941, Schweizer Druckund Verlagshaus.

34. West, C. E., Ritzgerald, C. R., and Sewell, J. H.: Cystoid macular edema following aphakic keratoplasty, Am. J. Ophthalmol. **75**:77, 1973.

35. Wolff, E.: Anatomy of the eye and orbit, ed. 6, Philadelphia, 1968, W. B. Saunders Co.

36. Wolff, E., and Penman, G. G.: The position occupied by the peripheral retinal fibres in the nerve fibre layer and at the nerve head. XVI Concilium Ophthalmologicum, Acta Lond. 1:625, 1950.

37. Worst, J. G. F.: Personal communication, 1974.

38. Yamada, E.: Some structural features of the fovea centralis in the human retina, Arch. Ophthalmol. 82:151, 1969.

39. Zinn, J. G.: Descriptio anatomica oculi humani iconibus illustrata, Göttingen, 1755, Abrami Vanderhoeck.

5

History of vitrectomy

A personal experience

DAVID KASNER

During the years 1962 to 1970, the open sky vitrectomy technique through a corneolimbal incision was successfully used for several indications:

1. Trauma
2. Cataract vitreous loss
3. Persistent hyperplastic primary vitreous
4. Amyloidosis
5. Aphakic corneal transplants
6. Nonmagnetic foreign bodies
7. Dislocated lenses
8. Old vitreous hemorrhage
9. Massive vitreous retraction
10. Postoperative complications
    a. Large iris prolapse
    b. Corneal edema due to vitreous touch
    c. Wound dehiscence
    d. Vitreous loss after suture removal
    e. Vitreous wick syndrome
    f. Persistent pupillary block with secondary glaucoma

One condition that constantly eluded successful treatment in my hands was diabetic retinitis proliferans; however, Dr. John Scott of Cambridge, England, has reported success using the corneal trephine opening approach.

During all these years I used three instruments: scissors, forceps, and Weck sponges. Deep in the vitreous cavity, the Weck sponges were cut down to 1×1×5 mm so as not to rub the iris on passing through the pupil. This helped reduce postoperative inflammation. I also tried hyaluronidase, thinking the enzyme would loosen and liquefy the vitreous. I thought it worked at first, but it really did not. The dense collagen cortex still had to be worked on mechanically with forceps and a sponge.

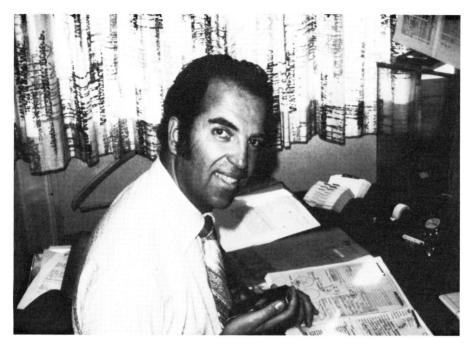

Fig. 5-1. Robert Machemer, M.D., who first developed the prototype of the VISC in 1969.

From 1966 to 1969, Dr. Robert Machemer was busy with retinal research but he observed vitrectomy from the corner of his eye (Fig. 5-1). In 1969 he deliberately set out to improve the tools used in vitreous surgery at the Bascom Palmer Eye Institute. He struck upon the idea of using a spiral drill inside a tubelike sleeve. In his garage, using a home-repair drill, he tested his idea on a raw egg; and it worked (Fig. 5-2). The contents of the egg were carried up and out over the top of the cylindrical sleeve without suction. To this he added suction for better control and, finally, a tube to infuse the eye with saline; thus was born the vitreous infusion suction cutter, or VISC.

The first few human eyes operated on after successful experiments with rabbits were done open sky. Then, in order not to sacrifice clear lenses, Dr. Machemer went through the pars plana. He later abandoned the drill concept and made improvements to reach the present design of the cutting tip. To this he added the fiber-optic light. During the same period other men—Douvas, Peyman, O'Malley, Witmer, Kloti—were working on machines of various designs.

Indications for the use of the machines gradually built up. In amyloidosis the clear lens was not sacrificed, and 20/20 to 20/30 phakic vision was achieved. With the open sky technique all eyes were made aphakic, and the anterior segments took a terrific beating. The same with old vitreous hemorrhage; but even more significant was the repeated success in diabetic retinitis proliferans. Finally, all the indications listed for the open sky technique became those for the pars plana approach.

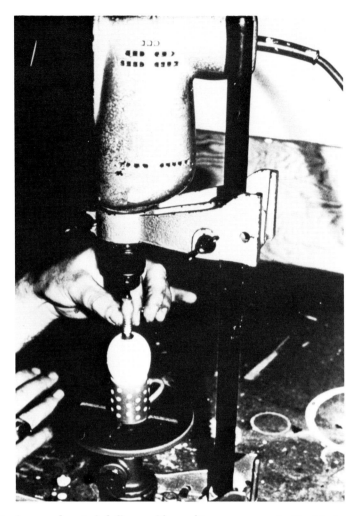

Fig. 5-2. The homemade spiral drill assembly working on an egg in Dr. Machemer's garage, which proved the notion that vitrectomy was possible with relatively simple instrumentation.

When I think back to the 1960's, however, when the open sky technique was riding high, a dense pupillary traumatic membrane was a simple problem. You merely had to open the eye, cut out the membrane, and clean out the vitreous. As an extra dividend you could better see the pathophysiology of trauma. I have sadly learned that the VISC cannot cut out some dense white membranes. Despite the obvious value of the VISC, I wonder at times whether the need for the open sky technique is really over and what the limits for the VISC and the other vitrectomy machines are.

6

Preoperative evaluation of patients for vitreous surgery

RONALD G. MICHELS
STEPHAN J. RYAN, Jr.

Patients considered for vitreous surgery require preoperative evaluation, including assessment of the ocular and medical status, and certain special tests. Vitreous surgery usually requires considerably longer operating time and is potentially more hazardous to the eye than many other ophthalmic surgical procedures. Also the results are less predictable. Therefore detailed preoperative evaluation is necessary to assist the surgeon in proper case selection, to plan details of the operation, and to permit realistic discussion with the patient of potential benefits and risks.

Preoperative evaluation includes a detailed ophthalmic and medical history and a complete examination of both eyes. Emphasis is placed on certain parts of the ocular physical examination, and a number of additional special tests may be required. Also particular attention is given to aspects of the patient's medical history; and a complete medical evaluation, including physical examination and laboratory tests, may be necessary before recommending vitreous surgery.

The concepts employed in vitreous surgery are still relatively new, and the cumulative experience of a number of surgeons will be necessary to further define the potential and limitations of this surgical procedure in various clinical situations. Careful preoperative evaluation and documentation are necessary to permit comparison of experience and results among surgeons.

OPHTHALMIC HISTORY

A complete ophthalmic history is obtained with emphasis on conditions currently affecting the eye. Specific aspects of the history depend on the underlying disease process. If surgery is contemplated for nonresolving vitreous opacities, the visual acuity and physical findings noted prior to the occurrence of opacities are important. Previous macular degeneration or traction retinal detachment involving the macula would preclude the possibility of good visual acuity even after successful vitrectomy; and this might influence the ophthalmologist not to recommend surgery if useful vision is present in the fellow eye. In diabetic patients a history of prior photocoagulation is important. The number and location of photocoagulation scars and areas of epiretinal proliferation are noted from prior records. Vitreoretinal adhesions are often present at sites of epiretinal proliferation, and special care is taken to avoid traction on these areas during surgery. Also we have the clinical impression that eyes previously treated by extensive photocoagulation tend to do especially well after vitrectomy.

The length of time the eye has been blind and any fluctuations in vision (including recent subjective improvement) are noted. Vitrectomy for vitreous opacities is considered if there is no evidence of clearing after 6 months and the fellow eye is also blind. Unless evidence of retinal detachment or other complications require earlier surgery, we wait a minimum of one year before considering vitrectomy if useful vision is present in the fellow eye. Vitreous hemorrhage of several years' duration is associated with some degree of ocular hemosiderosis. Even so, in our experience, vision may improve to a level as good as 20/30. Surgery is usually deferred if there has been significant recent visual improvement although opacities may have been present for a prolonged time.

Other conditions affecting the eye are noted, and the patient is specifically questioned regarding trauma and glaucoma. The possibility of a retained intraocular foreign body should not be overlooked; any penetrating injury may be associated with complex vitreoretinal relationships and complicated retinal detachment. History of glaucoma is important in planning the surgical procedure because intraocular pressure may be difficult to control postoperatively if loose blood remains in the eye or if sulfur hexafluoride (SF_6) gas is used and is not appropriately diluted with air. Details of prior operations are important if vitreous surgery is contemplated for complicated retinal detachment.

When the etiology of vitreous opacities is unknown, history is obtained regarding medical conditions affecting the eye. Diabetes mellitus with proliferative retinopathy is the most common cause of dense vitreous hemorrhage. Hemoglobin S/C disease should be considered in nondiabetic Negro patients; it may be associated with peripheral proliferative retinopathy and retinal detachment. Systemic hypertension may be associated with old retinal branch-vein obstruction, resulting in proliferative retinopathy and vitreous hemorrhage. Cellular infiltration of the vitreous may be the presenting sign of reticulum cell sarcoma in patients over 40 years of age, and history taking is directed toward detecting evidence of systemic involvement. A positive family history, combined with consistent vitreous opacities, may suggest the diagnosis of primary familial amyloidosis.

OPHTHALMIC EXAMINATION

Both eyes are carefully examined with methods including best corrected visual acuity, external evaluation, tonometry, slit lamp and fundus assessment, gonioscopy, and visual field testing. Special emphasis is placed on certain significant observations. When vision is less than 1/200, the presence of light-perception, shadow-motion, or hand-motion vision is determined and measured at the farthest distance perceived by the patient. Light projection is evaluated in each quadrant, and both the accuracy and the rapidity of subjective responses are recorded. In our experience the presence of brisk accurate light projection and the ability to accurately fixate a light are the most significant tests correlating favorably with visual improvement after vitrectomy in eyes with vitreous opacities. Two-point discrimination, color perception (red and green), and Maddox rod orientation are also tested. When these tests are positive, they suggest that the retina is capable of significant visual function. A negative response may be due merely to dense vitreous opacities. These tests, however, are usually uncertain in predicting the potential level of retinal function. Similarly, in our experience, tests for the presence of entoptic phenomena (angioscotomas) have not been useful in eyes with vitreous opacities.

External examination includes emphasis on testing muscle balance and pupillary responses. A large-angle horizontal tropia or any measurable vertical imbalance is likely to prevent fusion postoperatively—an important consideration if surgery is contemplated to achieve binocular function. Muscle imbalance is usually ignored if the fellow eye is blind, but inquiries about long-standing strabismus should be made and the possibility of amblyopia in one eye considered. Similarly congenital nystagmus is associated with a limited potential for distance vision, although we have observed pendular nystagmus to disappear in some cases after successful vitrectomy that resulted in visual improvement. Brisk pupillary response to direct light is a good prognostic sign. Pupillary responses are often sluggish in patients with proliferative diabetic retinopathy, however, and dense vitreous hemorrhage can cause complete loss of pupillary response to direct light. Also a significant afferent pupillary defect in one eye when compared to the fellow eye (Marcus Gunn pupil) is sometimes seen with dense vitreous opacities and in eyes which have clear media and total retinal detachment. Therefore such a pupillary defect does not indicate the anatomic status or functional capability of the retina. Size of the pupil after maximum dilatation is noted, and sphincterotomy or optical iridectomy may be necessary if the pupil cannot be dilated to more than 4 mm.

Slit lamp examination should include careful attention to the cornea, iris, lens, and vitreous cavity. Transient corneal edema often occurs after vitrectomy in aphakic eyes and tends to persist longer in diabetic patients. Endothelial guttatae or preoperative corneal edema may be associated with prolonged corneal decompensation after surgery. The iris is carefully examined before dilatation for evidence of new blood vessels (rubeosis), and the anterior chamber angle is examined by gonioscopy. New vessels are first seen along the pupillary margin and in the anterior chamber angle and may be easily overlooked. Rubeosis iridis causing secondary glaucoma or intraocular hemorrhage is the most common severe postoperative complication following otherwise successful vitrectomy in diabetic patients. When present preoperatively, definite rubeosis increases the likelihood of severe postoperative complications; in fact, some surgeons consider rubeosis iridis to be a contraindication to vitreous surgery.

If lens removal is anticipated as a part of the operation, the lens is examined— with emphasis on estimating the degree of nuclear sclerosis. Usually a lens demonstrating no more than 1+ (out of 4) nuclear sclerosis in patients less than 40 years of age can be easily removed by mechanical fragmentation and aspiration using the vitrectomy instrument. In patients over 40 years of age with nuclear sclerosis ranging from 1+ to 3+, the lens is softened by ultrasonic emulsification before being aspirated by the vitrectomy instrument. When marked nuclear sclerosis is present, the lens should be removed by conventional intra-capsular technique prior to or during the vitrectomy procedure.

If the media are sufficiently clear to permit visualization, the vitreous cavity and retina are examined by slit lamp (contact lens) biomicroscopy and in-direct ophthalmoscopy. Three-dimensional relationships of the vitreous and retina can be recorded on special charts designed to show both cross-sectional views of the vitreous cavity and a conventional drawing of the fundus. The position and density of transvitreal bands and sheets are recorded, with emphasis on areas of vitreoretinal adhesion, vitreous traction, and retinal detachment. The mechanical objective of vitrectomy is to relieve all vitreous traction on the ret-ina. Preoperative assessment of vitreoretinal relationships permits detailed plan-ning of the operation so the procedure can be performed with minimal traction on areas of vitreoretinal adhesion.

When vitreous opacities are present, visualization of the retina may be lim-ited or impossible. The vitreous is examined by indirect ophthalmoscopy, and certain structural features may be visible. The vitreous often has a funnel-like configuration, with the posterior hyaloid being separated from the retina and extending from the vitreous base anteriorly to the optic nerve and areas of proliferative retinopathy posteriorly. The examiner notes the presence of blood behind the posterior hyaloid and any elevated new blood vessels which may require endodiathermy during the vitrectomy procedure.

Dense opacities in the retrolenticular space may obstruct all visualization of the posterior vitreous cavity and retina. If this opaque vitreous moves freely with motion of the eye, it is usually easy to remove without fear of damaging the lens. If an opaque sheet is in contact with the lens and does not move with motion of the eye, however, special care is required when excising this sheet to avoid lens damage. The instrument tip is placed posterior to the opaque sheet, and moderate suction is applied to separate the sheet from the posterior lens capsule and bring it to the cutting port without causing distortion of the lens. In patients with dense opacities in the anterior vitreous, structural features of the vitreous cavity are determined during surgery as the opacities are being removed and the vitreous architecture is examined using fiber-optic intraocular il-lumination.

In eyes with moderately dense vitreous opacities, the examiner may be able

to visualize portions of the peripheral retina preoperatively by indirect ophthalmoscopy with scleral depression. This examination is important to determine
whether total retinal detachment is present, because retinal detachment significantly increases the difficulty and risk of complications during surgery. Also
transillumination is performed in eyes which have dense lens or vitreous opacities
to determine whether a pigmented mass lesion is present. Malignant melanoma
of the choroid may cause vitreous hemorrhage, and any transillumination defect
is evaluated further by ultrasound techniques.

Careful examination of the fellow eye is important in several respects. When
the etiology of vitreous opacities is unknown, the presence of a similar process
involving the fellow eye may aid in diagnosis of the underlying disease. Such
conditions as diabetic retinopathy, sickle cell retinopathy, periphlebitis, and severe hypertensive changes in the fellow eye suggest the cause of an existing
vitreous hemorrhage. Also the extent of retinal disease is often similar in both
eyes of a patient, and observations in the fellow eye may suggest what retinal
changes will be encountered after removal of vitreous opacities. Finally, the
visual prognosis of the fellow eye is important in deciding whether or not to
advise vitreous surgery. When vision in the fellow eye is threatened, as by
severe proliferative diabetic retinopathy, we may advise vitrectomy after only
6 months of nonresolving vitreous hemorrhage to determine whether the blind
eye can be visually rehabilitated before vision is lost in the fellow eye.

SPECIAL OPHTHALMIC TESTS

Additional tests including combined A- and B-scan ultrasonography and electroretinography (ERG) are valuable in the preoperative evaluation of certain
patients being considered for vitreous surgery. Radiographic examination of the
orbit is performed if a retained intraocular foreign body is suspected. External,
slit lamp, and fundus photography is used to document the preoperative appearance of the eye.

Ultrasound examination is valuable in eyes with opaque media to study
structural features in the vitreous cavity, to search for possible mass lesions,
and to assist in determining the presence and extent of retinal detachment. We
prefer combined A- and B-scan techniques, which provide a cross-sectional view
of the eye by B-scan and simultaneously demonstrate the amplitude of each
acoustic interface by A-scan display. Dense vitreous sheets, sites of vitreoretinal
adhesion, and areas of localized retinal detachment can often be demonstrated.
A question of major preoperative importance, however, is whether total retinal
detachment is present; and a detached retina is difficult to differentiate by A-
and B-scan from a detached thickened posterior hyaloid. The latter may have
a funnellike configuration extending from the vitreous base to the optic nerve
and may demonstrate morphologic features and acoustic impedance density identical to those of detached retina. Ultrasound observation of motion of the membrane after eye movement (kinetic scan) may help to differentiate between these
conditions. Also a combination of ultrasound and ERG testing may be useful.

EDITOR'S NOTE

Although some ultrasonographers believe they can clearly differentiate organized vitreous bands or detached posterior hyaloids from retinal detachment, I would personally agree with Dr. Michels and Dr. Ryan in advocating caution in the strict A- or B- or combined ultrasonic interpretation of these findings. There is little question that in some instances ultrasonic differentiation alone is almost impossible.

The ERG response to conventional light-flash stimuli may be markedly decreased or rendered unrecordable because of the filtering effect of the dense vitreous opacities. The recordable ERG response can be increased, however, by using a brighter stimulus flash (bright-flash ERG). This bright-flash stimulus has not been standardized among institutions, but it is generally applied in steps ranging from two to 1,000 times brighter than the brightest conventional ERG light-flash stimulus. The ERG response eventually reaches a maximum amplitude as brighter stimuli are used, and it begins to decrease if the stimulus flash is increased further. Often the B-wave amplitude is markedly decreased in eyes of diabetic patients; a deep A-wave may be recordable, and vision may improve after the vitreous opacities have been removed. Also an ERG response cannot be recorded in eyes with total retinal detachment, even when the media are clear; therefore a recordable bright-flash ERG response in eyes with vitreous opacities indicates that the retina is not totally detached and thus differentiates between retinal detachment and the funnellike vitreous configuration demonstrated by ultrasound examination.

Fluorescein angiography of the iris may become an important preoperative test in diabetic patients. As indicated previously, rubeosis iridis is a major cause of postoperative complications. If iris neovascularization is present preoperatively, the prognosis for successful surgery is decreased. Although experience with iris fluorescein angiography is limited, the technique may provide a method to identify preoperative iris neovascularization in eyes with subclinical findings; and it may help to document the course of postoperative changes, which could result in improved case selection and also provide additional information regarding the pathogenesis of this process.

MEDICAL EVALUATION

Medical evaluation includes history, physical examination, and certain laboratory tests directed toward predicting whether the patient can safely tolerate the operative procedure and associated anesthesia. The patient's life expectancy is important when considering vitreous surgery in diabetic patients with severe renal disease or other systemic complications. Both the physical condition and the psychologic status of the patient are evaluated; and consultation with the physician or internist treating the patient, and occasionally psychiatric evaluation, may be necessary.

Life expectancy of one to two years and a fifty-fifty chance of significant visual improvement are usually required before recommending vitreous surgery. When vision is profoundly reduced in both eyes, however, and ophthalmic evaluation indicates a high chance of visual improvement after surgery, we often recommend a vitrectomy without regard to the life expectancy—unless the operation would be a major threat to the patient's medical status. Improved vision may actually increase the life expectancy by permitting a diabetic patient to prepare and administer insulin at home. The ability to administer insulin is a requirement for entering home renal dialysis programs in some centers. Also improved vision may have a favorable effect on the patient's psychologic status and may result in improved compliance with medication and other therapeutic regimes.

History, physical examination, and laboratory tests are directed toward evaluating the cardiovascular system and renal status. Symptomatic coronary insufficiency or previous myocardial infarction may be indicated by history or ECG changes. A gallop heart rhythm and dependent or pulmonary edema indicate significant congestive heart failure. Elevated serum urea nitrogen (SUN) or creatinine levels associated with normochromic anemia indicate chronic renal failure. The cardiovascular status is important in determining the choice of local or general anesthesia and in estimating the degree of systemic risk associated with the operation. The renal status is important in estimating the life expectancy in certain diabetic patients.

Preference between local and general anesthesia for vitreous surgery varies from center to center; and, in addition, it is dependent on the medical status of the patient. Although the patient may be given the option of having either a local or a general anesthetic, in most cases we prefer general anesthesia for vitreous surgery. Patients with significant congestive heart failure or severe arrhythmias are poor risks for both local and general anesthesia. Every effort is made to improve the cardiovascular status before surgery. Local anesthesia is preferred for patients with systemic hypertension that is difficult to control or symptomatic coronary insufficiency. In these cases an intravenous infusion line is maintained, and an anesthesiologist is in attendance throughout the procedure. Severe azotemia and electrolyte imbalance, especially with high serum potassium levels, can often be improved by renal dialysis prior to vitreous surgery.

SUMMARY

History, physical examination, and special tests usually provide adequate information regarding the pathogenesis and current state of vitreoretinal pathology in patients being evaluated for vitreous surgery. An experienced surgeon can predict whether opacities will be readily removable and what structural alterations can be achieved by surgery; unfortunately the level of potential visual function often cannot be predicted by preoperative evaluation.

The ocular findings and visual needs of each patient are considered when the decision is being made whether to recommend vitreous surgery. Usually surgery is advised if both eyes are blind and the operation provides reasonable hope of some visual improvement. When good vision is present in the fellow eye, vitreous surgery is reserved for patients who have an especially favorable prognosis for achieving binocular function or who would otherwise develop further complications and progress to a permanently blind and inoperable state. In the latter situation surgery may be attempted to salvage a "spare tire" eye. Although successful vitrectomy may prevent subsequent destructive vitreous changes in certain eyes with proliferative diabetic retinopathy or following penetrating injuries of the posterior segment, we do not generally use vitreous surgery in eyes with good vision.

The preoperative findings, recommendation regarding surgery, and potential risks and benefits are discussed in detail with the patient. Though pars plana vitreous surgery is no longer experimental, the risk of complications with this procedure is still greater and the results more uncertain than with most other ophthalmic surgical procedures. The patient should understand that lens removal may be necessary as a part of the operation and that retinal detachment or other complications may occur and require further surgery or result in loss of all vision in the operated eye. Also the patient should understand that, despite successful vitrectomy, the underlying disease process is often not cured and retinal changes may progress and eventually result in further loss of vision. In effect, the patient should be aware of the many uncertainties related to the underlying disease process and this surgical procedure before he accepts a recommendation for pars plana vitreous surgery.

7

Ultrasonic evaluation of the vitreous

D. JACKSON COLEMAN

Opacification of the ocular media resulting from vitreous hemorrhage prevents adequate visual evaluation of the interior of the globe. Ultrasonography can portray both the extent of hemorrhagic changes and the intraocular pathology—e.g., retinal detachment, ocular tumor, intraocular foreign body—that may be obscured by the hemorrhage. In the preoperative evaluation of patients for vitrectomy, a differentiation (based on topographic configuration and amplitude patterns) may be reliably made among diffuse and organized hemorrhage, vitreous membranes, and retinal detachment. This graphic portrayal of the extent of hemorrhage, as well as coexisting ocular pathology, allows the vitreous surgeon to proceed in a more knowledgeable manner.

DISPLAY MODES

There are three basic display modes currently used in ophthalmic ultrasound: A-, B-, and M-mode. Of these three, B-mode is the most easily interpreted by the ophthalmologist because of its topographic cross-sectional presentation, which is very similar to a histologic section. The A- and M-modes provide specific echo amplitude and pulsatile characteristics respectively. A combined examination technique using B-mode to localize and characterize the intraocular abnormality[2,4,10] and A-mode to specify its amplitude characteristics[8-10] has proved to be most helpful in determining the nature of these abnormalities. M-mode is utilized when knowledge of the pulsatile nature (whether vascular or magneto-kinetic) of the abnormality is required.

A-mode

A-mode uses a fixed probe that directs the sound beam along a single axis of the eye. The reflections returning from the ocular structures to the transducer are displayed on an oscilloscope, and the height of these echoes corresponds to the amount of sound energy reflected from the ocular structure. The amplitude

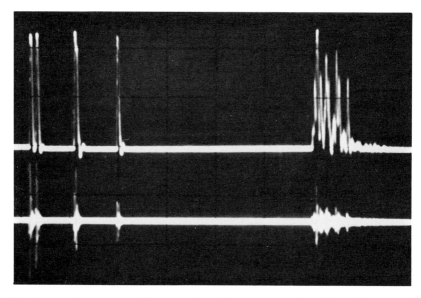

Fig. 7-1. A-scan ultrasonogram of a normal eye demonstrating the echo configuration obtained in an axial plane. The characteristic axial A-scan consists of two initial echo spikes produced by the cornea, echoes from the anterior and posterior lens capsules, and the acoustically quiet zone of the vitreous followed by echoes from the retina, choroid, and sclera. The echoes from the retrobulbar fat gradually diminish to the base line.

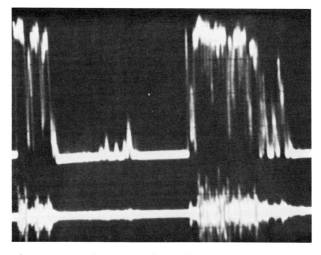

Fig. 7-2. A-scan ultrasonogram of a vitreous hemorrhage showing the low-to-moderate–amplitude echoes within the vitreous compartment. These echoes do not characteristically approach the height of the retinal echo, a feature more readily demonstrated on the videotrace (top) than on the radio-frequency trace (bottom).

of the echo not only is dependent on the orientation of the beam but is also related to the difference in the acoustic impedance at the tissue boundary. A-mode may be presented as a "video envelope" of the specific reflections and/or the original bipolar response of the transducer to the received echoes (radio-frequency trace).

The A-scan display of a normal eye is shown in Fig. 7-1. In the typical axial A-scan, high-amplitude echoes are produced by the two surfaces of the cornea and by the anterior and posterior lens capsules; the vitreous is represented by an interval with no echoes above base line; and it is followed by the complex of echoes from the retina, choroid, sclera, and retrobulbar fat.

Of primary interest in the present discussion is the area of the vitreous, which is normally nonreflecting (called an acoustic quiet zone). Like the lens the vitreous is a homogeneous structure which presents no reflecting surfaces. The appearance of echoes in this normally sonolucent area (Fig. 7-2) is an indication of an ocular abnormality, and the differentiation of vitreous pathology is based on the echo variation observed—for example, from a detached retina the echo is higher than from a vitreous membrane.

Measurement of the vitreous compartment is often of use to the diagnostician and can be obtained with ultrasonographic techniques. Tissue thickness of 0.2 mm may be delineated using high-frequency (20 MHz) A-scan methods. A tissue separation of at least 0.2 mm is required to allow the echo from a structure such as the anterior cornea to return to base line so that a subsequent echo spike unmarred by decay from the previous signal can be identified. In vitreous surgery, measurements are useful in determining the distance between membranes and the retina and in localizing foreign bodies.

B-mode

In B-scan ultrasonography the display is observed on an oscilloscope which is slaved to the movement of the transducer. The echo spikes of the A-scan are presented as brightness-modulated dots to form the B-scan. As the transducer is moved, these dots connect—producing a two-dimensional outline or a cross section of the eye (Fig. 7-3). The two surfaces of the cornea can be delineated, followed by the sonolucent area of the anterior chamber. The anterior lens capsule is usually lost in the echo complex of the iris, but the posterior lens capsule may be well demonstrated. As just described in the discussion of A-mode, the vitreous cavity is normally sonolucent because of its homogeneous composition. The retina, choroid, and sclera are represented by a high-amplitude (bright) concave structure preceding the crescent-shaped retrobulbar echo pattern, which may be indented by the V-shaped notch produced by the optic nerve.

The presence of echoes in the normally clear vitreous cavity indicates the position and extent of hemorrhage, fibrin, or membrane (Fig. 7-4).

In most B scan displays the equatorial regions of both the lens and the globe do not lie parallel to the examining beam and are therefore poorly depicted. These equatorial regions may be brought into view by adjusting the transducer

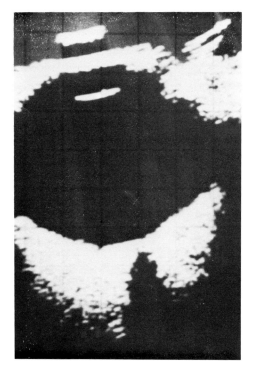 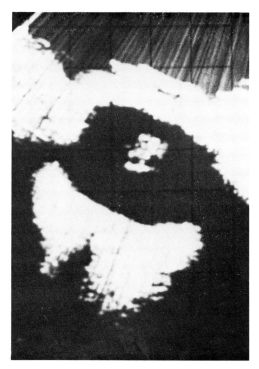

Fig. 7-3   Fig. 7-4

Fig. 7-3. B-scan ultrasonogram of a normal eye taken in an axial plane in which the two surfaces of the cornea, the anterior and posterior lens capsules, and the concave curvature of the vitreoretinal interface may be seen. The anterior chamber, interior of the lens, and vitreous compartment all appear sonolucent due to their homogeneous structure.

Fig. 7-4. B-scan ultrasonogram of a vitreous hemorrhage appearing as a moderately dense isolated coagulum in midvitreous.

orientation to the globe or by having the patient alter his direction of gaze (thereby changing the globe's orientation to the transducer).

M-mode

The M-mode, which shows motion of tissues, uses amplitude-modulated dots on an oscilloscope.[7] Any movement of a tissue surface causes the representative line of dots to wiggle accordingly, and the amount of tissue response to any induced force can be judged. In vitreous surgery the M-mode is most useful in demonstrating the movement of ferrous foreign bodies in a magnetic field.

TECHNIQUES

In our laboratory the immersion method of ultrasonography is preferred[3] since it allows better resolution of the anterior segment, variation of the transducer frequency during examination, and consecutive serial sectioning of the eye and orbit. In our system it also permits simultaneous monitoring of the A- and B-

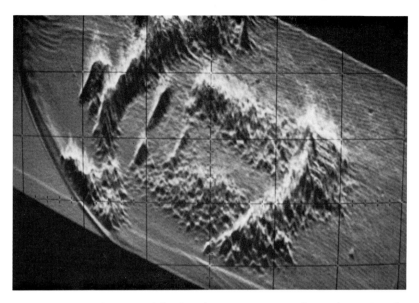

Fig. 7-5. Isometric three-dimensional display of a massive vitreous hemorrhage. A cyclitic membrane posterior to the lens obscured visual evaluation. The comparative echo height information available on this type of display is evident from the echoes in midvitreous, which do not approach the posterior lens height or the retinal surface. The scan can be rotated through 360° and viewed from different angles of perspective.

scans. We feel that these advantages far outweigh the drawbacks of the technique—the additional effort required for patient preparation.

Contact B-scan equipment[1] is also available, is relatively inexpensive, and has the distinct advantage of portability. Contact scan techniques, however, do not allow a high degree of resolution of the anterior ocular structures or the penetration into the orbit obtained with a water bath standoff; but they do permit good evaluation of the vitreous compartment.

Besides the conventional method of viewing ultrasonograms (i.e., by visually comparing the B-scan display and the A-scan echo amplitude through a particular horizontal or vertical plane), more informative display techniques may be employed.

Color coding[5] can be used to improve the amount of gray scale (i.e., the amplitude information on the two-dimensional B-mode picture). This feature may help distinguish membranes or retina in relation to lower-amplitude fibrin. A new technique called isometric viewing,[6] which is a three-dimensional portrayal, can also be implemented. On this type of display, the two dimensions of the B-scan are still present and the amplitude spikes of the A-mode display become the third dimension.

Fig. 7-5 shows the isometric display of an ultrasonogram of a patient with vitreous hemorrhage. The height of echoes in midvitreous and the cross-sectional dimensions of the hemorrhage are simultaneously displayed. This three-dimensional image can be viewed from different angles, an option which is particularly useful in planning vitreous surgery since the surgeon can better perceive the intravitreal relationships and can thus gain a mental grasp of intraocular pathology nearly as vivid as by direct visualization. This information can be obtained by simultaneously observing the A- and B-scans; therefore the new display technique does not provide greater information but rather a far better means of analyzing it.

Kinetic scans, obtained by having the patient move his eye from side to side while fast-sector scanning is performed, allow the examiner to observe the relative mobility of intraocular pathology and to determine the attachments of vitreous hemorrhage to the ocular walls. When the vitreous hemorrhage is unrestrained by membrane formation, it can be seen on kinetic scanning to flow freely and in most instances to settle inferiorly due to gravitational forces.

Since hemorrhage into the fluid vitreous moves freely and hemorrhage into the solid vitreous exhibits a more damped movement, any observed hemorrhage may by inference be localized to the solid or fluid vitreous by this method.

ULTRASONIC DIAGNOSIS OF VITREOUS HEMORRHAGE

In many cases of vitreous hemorrhage, no visualization of the interior of the eye is possible; thus ultrasonography provides the only information as to the density, extent of hemorrhage, and morphologic retinal status. Often the source of bleeding can be identified, particularly in younger patients, with solid vitreous, in whom bleeding or disruption of the vitreous can be traced to the globe wall. Organization of hemorrhage into membranes, as well as associated ocular changes such as lens dislocation or retinal detachment, can be shown.

Light diffuse vitreous hemorrhage usually presents no discrete acoustic interfaces and thus will appear sonolucent. When the hemorrhage has coagulated, the acoustic picture may range from scattered low-amplitude echoes to dense aggregates of echoes—corresponding to the density of the clots. In the final stages of organization, vitreous membranes can be identified as linear configurations.

Fig. 7-6 shows the ultrasonogram of a patient with light-perception vision. A diaphenous vitreous membrane of the type that is likely to clear spontaneously is noted posterior to the lens. In cases such as this, ultrasound may be instrumental in determining the feasibility of observing the patient for a longer period of time.

A membrane stretching across midvitreous with attachments slightly anterior to the ora serrata is shown in Fig. 7-7. Multiple serial sections showed no attachment of this membrane to the optic nerve head, and the pattern was interpreted as a vitreous veil. The case underscores the importance of obtaining a complete topographic picture with serial sections and determining the points of attachment of any membrane to the region of both the ora serrata and the disc. Detached retina will always insert at these two locations, and only rarely will a membrane mimic retinal detachment in both amplitude and such a unique morphologic pattern.

When vitreous hemorrhage or membranes exist concurrently with retinal de-

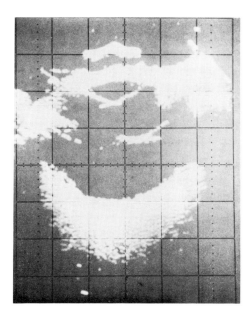 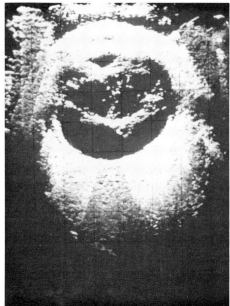

Fig. 7-6   Fig. 7-7

Fig. 7-6. B-scan ultrasonogram of a vitreous membrane that stretches across the globe with points of attachment slightly posterior to the ora serrata. The variations in membrane thickness are typical and aid in differentiation from retina.

Fig. 7-7. B-scan ultrasonogram of a vitreous veil stretching across the globe with attachments slightly anterior to the ora serrata. This membrane did not attach to the optic nerve head.

tachment, as shown in Fig. 7-8, *A*, the additional information available from the A-scan (Fig. 7-8, *B*) is of assistance in differentiating these two conditions. Retinal echoes are usually equal in height to the echoes from the posterior scleral wall; diffuse hemorrhage or membranes do not generally produce reflections of this amplitude. When a gray scale component is available on the B-scan, the comparative echo amplitude should be apparent to the examiner. In the absence of adequate gray scale, the A-scan should be constantly monitored to determine the relative echo height of intraocular pathology.

The area of greatest diagnostic difficulty is the distinction of proliferative membranes from detached retina. Membranes resulting from diabetic retinopathy most typically emanate from the regions of the optic disc and macula. Their topographic configuration may therefore mimic the appearance of a posterior pole traction detachment (Fig. 7-9). High-amplitude echoes can be produced by both proliferans and retina, so comparative A-scan analysis may not contribute to differentiation.

We have found that subtle acoustic characteristics of proliferative membranes may be of assistance in identifying the membrane. In general, proliferative membranes emanating from the posterior pole do not extend beyond midvitreous and

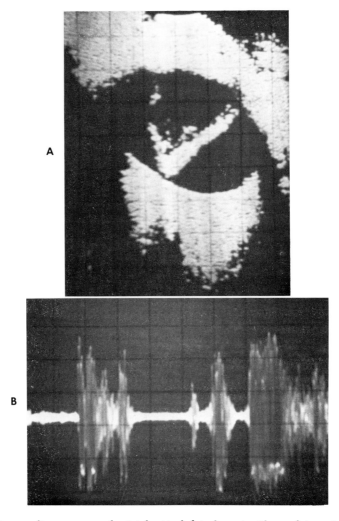

Fig. 7-8. **A,** B-scan ultrasonogram of a total retinal detachment with overlying vitreous hemorrhage. The retina is identified as a high-amplitude membrane extending from the optic nerve to the ora serrata. **B,** A-scan ultrasonogram of **A** demonstrating the comparative echo heights on a radio-frequency trace. The moderate-amplitude reflections from hemorrhage precede the echoes from the retina, which approximate the height of the scleral echoes.

thus cannot be traced to an attachment site at the ora serrata. On kinetic scanning they may be seen to move freely, in contrast to the more restrained movement of detached retina. Though the echo amplitude of proliferative membranes may be very similar to that of retina in one scan plane, rotating the scanner arm 180° may indicate an inconsistent thickness of the membranes and thus differentiate them from retina (which maintains a uniform thickness in all meridians).

It must be emphasized, however, that absolute differentiation of membrane and retina cannot be made in all cases. Nevertheless, the presence of prolifer-

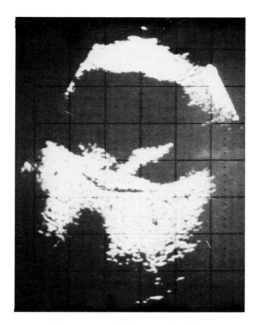

Fig. 7-9. B-scan ultrasonogram of retinitis proliferans. This characteristic pattern demonstrates dense high-amplitude membranes confined to the posterior compartment of the vitreous.

ative membranes and their localization can prepare the surgeon for vascular membranes or retina in this area.

ULTRASONIC EVALUATION OF TRAUMA

Since ocular trauma usually results in immediate opacification of the ocular media, ultrasound is essential in evaluating the traumatized eye. In addition to showing the hemorrhagic vitreal abnormalities already described as identifiable, ultrasound can localize and quantify conditions uniquely associated with trauma—e.g., the localization of a posterior perforation site, a dislocated lens, or an intraocular foreign body and the determination of the magnetic properties of a foreign body.

The information available from ultrasonic examination may direct management of the traumatized eye. Many patients present with such severe ocular changes that conventional methods of observation and medication might impede rather than speed visual recovery. Ultrasonic assessment of the severity of hemorrhage and associated ocular changes (e.g., retinal detachment) aids the surgeon in selecting the appropriate candidates for surgery, the timing of surgery, and the proper surgical procedure.

Traumatic changes presenting with such a poor prognosis that surgical intervention is required include the following:

1. Ruptured posterior lens capsule
2. Ciliary body laceration extending to the retina and/or double perforations involving the retina

3. Retained reactive foreign body
4. Massive vitreous hemorrhage with retinal detachment

The topographic capabilities of the B-scan are necessary to delineate the posterior lens capsule and to detect a dehiscence representing posterior capsule rupture as shown in Fig. 7-10. Anterior vitreal reaction to the dispersed lens material can also be seen in this particular case.

In younger individuals, with solid vitreous, the track of vitreous hemorrhage is more easily identified. When attempting to localize a posterior perforation site, the surgeon may find this fact important. Ultrasound cannot reliably indicate the site of a scleral rupture; but by tracing a path of hemorrhage through the vitreous compartment from an anterior injury to a point of attachment at the posterior globe wall, the surgeon can surmise a posterior perforation site. A lacerating injury that has not perforated the posterior wall of the globe will generally demonstrate a more contained area of hemorrhage. The localization of a posterior perforation site can indicate to the surgeon the site of his incision and may eliminate undue exploration and pressure on a traumatized eye.

The localization and characterization of small ocular or orbital foreign bodies (magnetic or nonmagnetic) can be a time-consuming and frustrating task. Therefore a thorough radiographic evaluation is best performed prior to ultrasonography. With this prior localization the examiner can devote his time to the characterization of the foreign body and the determination of its magnetic properties.

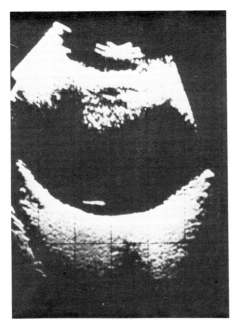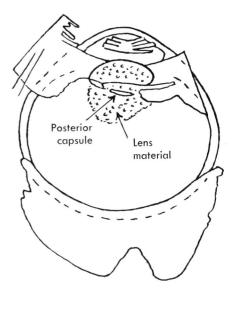

Posterior capsule

Lens material

Fig. 7-10. B-scan ultrasonogram of a rupture of the posterior lens capsule. The normally smooth high-amplitude contour of the capsule is no longer discernable acoustically. Lens material has been released into the anterior vitreous, producing a diffuse moderate-amplitude echo pattern in the anterior vitreous compartment.

The outline of a metal fragment surrounded by blood can be enhanced by lowering the sensitivity setting. Thus echoes from the blood (being of lower amplitude than echoes from the foreign body) will drop away. Since sound is transmitted through metal faster than through surrounding vitreous, the retina directly behind an intraocular foreign body may appear raised. This is an acoustic artifact and does not indicate retinal detachment. In addition, the absorption of sound by the foreign body may produce a shadowed area in the region posterior to the foreign body—which can be used as a pointer to indicate the location of a foreign body, even when it is embedded in the sclera or the retrobulbar fat.

A foreign body demonstrating these classic acoustic criteria is shown in Fig. 7-11.

The magnet test is used to determine the magnetic properties of a foreign body. In addition to determining the amount of magnetism inherent in a foreign body, by visually correlating the velocity of motion, the distance moved, and the amount of recoil, this method can determine how rigidly the foreign body is held by a hemorrhagic capsule within the vitreous. It is important to position the magnet well away from the eye, however, and to approach the eye lateral to the lens so the foreign body will not be accidentally pulled into the lens.

Fig. 7-12 shows the pulsatile properties of a magnetic foreign body, as documented on the M-mode, in the field of a Bronson-Magnion pulsed magnet.

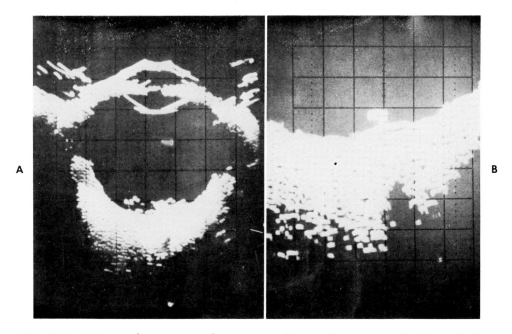

A **B**

Fig. 7-11. A, B-scan ultrasonogram of a traumatized eye with an intraocular foreign body. **B,** A portion of the posterior pole has been electronically expanded. In the expanded view a lower-sensitivity setting isolates the foreign body, which had been obscured by hemorrhage. An apparent elevation of the retinal surface and a notch in the retrobulbar fat pattern are both acoustic artifacts produced by the foreign body.

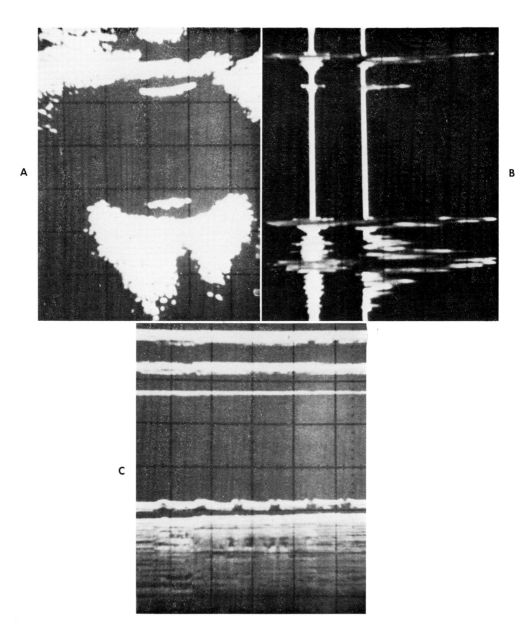

Fig. 7-12. Comparative B-, A-, and M-scans of an eye with a magnetic intraocular foreign body. The foreign body may be seen on the B-scan (**A**) as the sense echo preceding the retina and on the A-scan (**B**) as the very high-amplitude echo in the otherwise sonolucent vitreous cavity. On the M-scan (**C**) the response of the metal in a pulsed magnetic field is seen as fluctuations in the trace that precedes the retina/choroid/sclera complex.

A metal fragment as small as 0.2 mm can be identified ultrasonographically. Small metal and glass foreign bodies, however, may be missed if they are not oriented properly to the transducer. Vegetable foreign material is far more difficult to localize unless it is surrounded by some inflammatory reaction.

The ominous prognostic situation of retinal detachment with massive vitreous hemorrhage is distinguished by the identification of retinal leaves billowing into the vitreous compartment. In massive hemorrhage the configuration of coalesced blood and membranes may be so stratified that differentiation of small localized areas of detachment cannot be absolutely achieved. The overall definition of such extensive trauma, however, will usually be sufficient to indicate the proper management.

•   •   •

Ultrasound provides a unique ability to characterize vitreous opacities. The density and location of hemorrhage, and the presence of fibroproliferative membranes, retinal detachment, and occult tumors can be shown with ultrasound. In the preoperative evaluation of trauma, the extent of structural change can be evaluated and the surgical management of the injury more knowledgeably directed.

REFERENCES

1. Bronson, N.: Development of a simple B-scan ultrasonoscope, Trans. Am. Acad. Ophthalmol. Otolaryngol. **70**:365, 1972.
2. Coleman, D. J.: Ultrasound in vitreous surgery, Trans. Am. Acad. Ophthalmol. Otolaryngol. **76**:467, 1972.
3. Coleman, D. J.: Reliability of ocular and orbital diagnosis with B-scan ultrasound. Part I, Ocular diagnosis, Am. J. Ophthalmol. **73**:501, 1972.
4. Coleman, D. J., and Franzen, L. A.: Vitreous surgery: preoperative evaluation and prognostic value of ultrasonic display of vitreous hemorrhage, Arch. Ophthalmol. **92**:375, 1974.
5. Coleman, D. J., and Katz, L.: Color coding of B-scan ultrasonograms, Arch Ophthalmol. **91**:429, 1974.
6. Coleman, D. J., Katz, L., and Lizzi, F. L.: Isometric three-dimensional viewing of ultrasonograms, Arch. Ophthalmol. **93**:1362, 1975.
7. Coleman, D. J., and Weininger, R. B.: Ultrasonic M-mode technique in ophthalmology, Arch. Ophthalmol. **82**:475, 1969.
8. Ossoinig, K.: Clinical echo-ophthalmology. In Blodi, K. C., editor: Current concepts in ophthalmology, St. Louis, 1972, The C. V. Mosby Co., vol. 3.
9. Purnell, E.: Intensity modulated (B-scan) ultrasonography. In Goldberg, R., and Sarin, L., editors: Ultrasonics in ophthalmology, Philadelphia, 1967, W. B. Saunders Co.

Round table discussion

Chapters 1 to 7

McClure   What's the difference in vitrectomy when one uses a temporal or nasal entry into the globe? What do you do with some of the other vitrectomy equipment, like the O'Malley unit, that employs simultaneous entry into the eye of two instruments? Is an anterior limbal approach superior to the posterior pars plana approach?

Shields   I just made the point that the ciliary processes, especially on the nasal side, may be more elongated and may extend all the way into the ciliary crest. By doing one or two things, one can be sure he is not going through any significant ocular tissue. First of all, if the media is clear, you can look in and depress the pars plana. If there's no retina abnormally inserted anterior in that particular location, you're probably safe. If the media is opaque, you can transilluminate, see the ora serrata pretty well, and feel a little bit confident that you're not going through retina on that side.

   The point is that I didn't advocate placing the instrument in any specific area, but I did mention precaution when one cuts on the nasal side. In summary, indirect ophthalmoscopy and scleral depression or transillumination can help make certain that you're not going through an abnormal portion of retina when surgically entering the globe.

Jaffe   In PHPV, one of the things I've been impressed with, in the few cases I've done by an open sky technique, is that the amount of bleeding is relatively little. One of the reasons I like the anterior approach is, in the first place, I don't do the posterior approach, and I don't have any experience with it. So needless to say, I'm biased. One of the theoretical reasons I like it is that you can actually pick up the membrane and see what you're doing under the scope and section all around. We have a few stunning results of these, with movies, and reappearance of the fundus reflex.

Ryan   Dr. Jaffe made a good point, as we just discussed PHPV. And Dr. Shields pointed out how the retina can be drawn over to the region of the lens into that retrolenticular area; and because of that, I think if one is going to operate, it's worthwhile to go in by the anterior, specifically the limbal approach. We would use the Roto-Extractor to remove it but come from the anterior approach. I know I've argued with Ron Michels and a few others about just exactly how to approach that; but in point of fact, it was one of the Wilmer cases reported by Ron Smith and Dr. Maumenee in which inadvertently, after removing the lens, they cut the retina, as has been previously reported in the literature. So I think, to avoid a retinectomy anytime that one is concerned—whether it's because you're worried about choroidal effusion, a ciliary detachment, a retina drawing up in that area—you just have to approach it cautiously.

I think Dr. Shields pointed out also that the anatomy of the pars plana favors one going in temporally, specifically as one usually has about 1 mm more pars plana to work with temporally than nasally, and also the convenience of the surgeon, i.e., not having to go across the bridge of the nose. In point of fact, there are penetrating injuries temporally or other reasons that are certainly indications for entering the pars plana on its nasal side.

Peyman I don't have any experience with PHPV, but in cases where one wants to do a two-needle technique through the pars plana and use the nasal area, as a rule of thumb I go about 4 to 4.5 mm behind the limbus, and in that instance one is within the pars plana of the nasal area. In only one case out of more than 100, I had to go nasally because it was a retinal detachment and there was a distinct membrane temporally, and I went through the nasal area. In the two-needle techniques I usually go about 4 to 4.5 mm nasally with a needle through the pars plana, and I've not encountered any problems.

• • •

Cockerham What is meant by an early case, or the definition of early vitreous touch, and what time period is indicated for surgical intervention?

Jaffe I don't want to be dogmatic about this, so I will. In the first place, I call early vitreous touch, again meaning "adherence," only if it is associated with corneal edema. In other words, just don't intervene because the vitreous is against the cornea. You have to have evidence of corneal edema overlying this area. Early, to me, means 48 to 96 hours postoperatively. How long do you wait? I believe that if you're beginning to get decompensation of the cornea this is one of the true surgical emergencies. I'd try medical methods first, i.e., mydriatics and hyperosmotic agents. I might try it again 1 day later; and if it didn't work, I'd intercede by doing the Leahey treatment. You may save yourself a very serious type of procedure, like a penetrating keratoplasty.

So, as least in my own hands, if you're alert to this and you pick it up early and you don't sit on the egg for 7 to 21 days, you're much more likely to achieve a successful result. Again, there is no guarantee, and you may also have to associate this treatment with getting rid of the pupillary block, perhaps with an iridectomy or some other method of treating the associated pupillary block.

· · ·

McClure   We've had several questions about asteroid hyalosis. Would the panel consider removal of vitreous in cases of asteroid hyalosis if there was retinal detachment and the asteroid hyalosis prevented localization of the hole? Would the panel advocate vitrectomy if the asteroid prevented a fundus view for photocoagulation if that was needed?

Peyman   If a patient has a retinal detachment and one can't evaluate the fundus, as a matter of rule I always do a vitrectomy, regardless of if it is asteroid hyalosis or what other condition has existed that contributed to the vitreous hemorrhage. If I can't localize the tear and the vitreous is sufficiently cloudy, I regularly perform vitrectomy and then proceed with retinal detachment surgery.

Jaffe   I'd like not to get too much involved with that aspect. I would like to ask Ed Okun a question if I may. I recall reading in Paul Cibis' book that he did vitrectomies, if I am quoting it correctly, in three cases of asteroid hyalosis because it interfered with vision. As you know, I think the world of that book, and yet I have been looking for cases of asteroid hyalosis which actually significantly caused decreased vision, and I've never found one. I wonder if this is due to the fact that I just haven't found one and that others have. I'd like your opinion on it.

Okun   I think it's rare to find asteroid hyalosis affecting the patient's visual acuity, but it certainly can occur, particularly when the asteroid hyalosis is extremely close to the retina. I've seen where big balls have actually been directly over the macula when it is very close, and it can affect vision under those circumstances.

I recall performing a vitrectomy on one of the patients who had a liquid silicone injection to displace the asteroid hyalosis anteriorly. It wasn't actually entirely removed, and I don't think that patient had very much improvement in visual function. I'm not 100% certain of it.

With regard to whether one should always do a vitrectomy if one is having difficulty in visualizing a retinal detachment, I think you may end up doing a large number of vitrectomies in this situation. We've all seen patients who had vitreous hemorrhages and you have to really wait awhile for them to clear.

As a matter of fact, it's a very common history to have a patient seen with a vitreous hemorrhage and you can't see into that eye. Unfortunately they are often just told to go, rather than have an excellent examination or hospitalization and bilateral patches until you can find the break. Frequently we see them with enough visualization so you can do something about them. I think a time limit is needed, perhaps somewhere in the vicinity of a couple of months with absolutely no clearing or membrane formation, prior to consideration of vitrectomy. I only have two cases, out of all the vitrectomies we've done, that were done for the purpose of clearing what we felt was a rhegmatogenous detachment in order to go ahead with the surgery. Others may have different experiences along those lines.

Douvas I'd like to comment that in agreement with Dr. Jaffe, whom I can rarely disagree with, that my experience was that most cases of asteroid hyalosis, regardless of degree, have good visual acuity. Many times when it's a combination of hyalosis and cataract, you remove the cataract and this eye will get back 20/20 vision; yet they're so dense you wonder how they can see, but they do see quite well. I believe Troutman reported a case that improved from 20/200 to 20/30 following vitrectomy for apparently a very severe hyalosis.

Peyman I don't perform routine vitrectomies in all cases of hemorrhage combined with retinal detachment. I didn't mean fresh vitreous hemorrhage. I meant if vitreous hemorrhage was old enough and sufficient enough to impair vision.

Shields I've been impressed about one thing concerning asteroid hyalosis. We have seen a number of cases now (and I don't know whether this is in the literature or not) with a very high incidence of coexistent severe disciform macular degeneration. Sometimes the asteroid hyalosis can be quite dense and you can barely see the disciform lesion back there. In other cases it has been so dense that you couldn't see it, and you can pick it up then with B-scan ultrasound. If you have a patient with severe asteroid hyalosis and reduced vision, in which you can't see the fundus, don't attribute the visual decline to the asteroid hyalosis until you've at least done a B-scan ultrasound and looked for a disciform process back there. I personally think there's a higher incidence, in my own observation, of disciform macular degeneration in patients who have asteroid hyalosis.

Coleman I'd just like to disagree a little bit with the question of vitreous hemorrhage and retinal detachment. I'm not sure, Ed. In a rhegmatogenous detachment with a spontaneous bleed, I agree with you; but following trauma I've seen so many cases of severe vitritis with a retinal detachment that just get worse and worse. I think that following trauma with vitritis, you should go in and clear them and do the retina immediately rather than wait. Do we agree on that?

Okun A hundred percent. There's no question on trauma, and all I can do tomorrow is give some of the horrible results that have come about because of waiting on them. I think that possibly those traumatic hemorrhages will eventually clear; but by the time they clear, the fibrous membranes that are formed are so tough you can't do anything about them. So in cases of trauma, I definitely would agree to clear them early.

Peyman My experiences are also the same. I've done a few vitrectomies on old trauma and I found the retina was almost detached because of the development of retinal membranes, and it was almost impossible to put it back. In cases of penetrating injury I went ahead and did immediate vitrectomy and took care of the retinal injury immediately, and the results were much better.

• • •

McClure   In the case of a long (over a year) retained intraocular foreign body and siderosis bulbi including corneal involvement with iron, would the panel prefer (1) removal of the intraocular foreign body through the pars plana and use of a chelating agent to combat the siderosis or (2) remove the foreign body and do a vitrectomy to combat the continuous retinal damage from the heavy vitreous deposit of iron? Who'd like to tackle that?

Peyman   If a patient has an intraocular foreign body for over a year, this foreign body is usually encapsulated within a fibrous membrane or whatever, and vitreous opacities left there. It's almost impossible to remove the foreign body alone. I think the best approach is to combine a vitrectomy in order to actually remove these foreign bodies. It's not impossible to remove the foreign body and take the forceps and go and grasp it and bring it out, because this foreign body—and the material which is around this foreign body—has attachment to the vitreous base and other areas of the retina. I always do a vitrectomy in these cases; and if it's not a magnetic foreign body, then I remove the foreign body with a forceps. If it is a magnetic foreign body, then after vitrectomy, if the foreign body is a small one, I either suck it through the instrument or, if it's large enough, by a magnet. With regard to chelating agents, I have no experience with that.

Douvas   If it's a nonmagnetic foreign body, one year old, and fibrosed in and causing no problem, why not leave it?

Peyman   That depends upon where the foreign body is located, of course. If the foreign body is in the wall of the eye and you can see very well inside the eye, there's no reason to do anything. If the foreign body is inhibiting vision and by ultrasound you find the retina is on and other function tests are eventually indicating that some functioning retina exists, then I'd go ahead. Of course, the preop evaluation is very important.

Cockerham   I think there's a large number of eyes with retinal detachment that have opacification of the media that can be treated by going ahead with a buckle. I think the rule of thumb is that if you can see enough of the fundus to make a reasonably good guess and feel confident, you can reattach the retina.

• • •

Question   Dr. Jaffe, do you have any cases where air has caused further endothelial decompensation with the Leahey-type treatment?

Jaffe   That's an interesting question. It's very hard to state, in a case like this, whether it's just normal progression of decompensation or whether it's due to the air. I got a call about 4 months ago that said, "Did you see that paper where air is so destructive to the endothelium?" I didn't see the paper at that time, but I asked if the experiments had been done in rabbits and the answer was affirmative. I'm not so sure that air has a toxic effect on corneal endothelium—perhaps not in humans, even though some people have shown it in rabbits. It seems as though all experimental work done on rabbit's corneas seem to show, just like cancer in mice, everything you want it to show. Nevertheless, I haven't yet recognized that the air itself was responsible for this; and this may just be lack of clinical alertness on my part. I don't know.

Gitter I saw one adult, a 45-year-old patient who I thought had PHPV in which the lens was absent without a history of lens extraction. The lens capsule had apparently spontaneously ruptured early in life with resorption of lens cortical material, leaving the patient aphakic with remnants of PHPV and a quiet-looking eye and minimal microphthalmos (determined by time-amplitude ultrasonography) which amazed me. I thought about it then, and I've thought about it since; you just don't see adults with PHPV. Why is it?

Okun We probably don't see them in practice. Those eyes are probably not recognizable as having had that, or they are in the pathology lab. That is just my guess; I've never seen an adult.

Jaffe Usually when you do see an adult with PHPV with the eye still in the head, it's just one of the more minor forms of PHPV. Look, PHPV can go all the way from a Mittendorf dot to the full-blown syndrome that Dr. Shields discussed. I reviewed many pages in the vitreous reviews several years ago describing minor and major forms of PHPV. When you see an adult eye with what you think clinically has been PHPV, it's just one of the more minor forms of involvement. That is why the eye went on to adulthood. I don't think, with some of the eyes that you saw today—with the retina pulled right into the pre-retinal membrane, and with the perilenticular hemorrhages which occur, and the growth of the globe beginning to exceed the growth of the retrolental membrane—that these eyes are going to survive into adult life. At least, that's what I think.

· · ·

McClure Following a Kasner anterior vitrectomy, what is the incidence of prolonged corneal edema, of persistent uveitis, of hypotony, and phthisis bulbi?

Kasner I had thirty-five former residents who sent me the results of 105 cases of vitrectomy that they had performed for normal vitreous loss during cataract surgery. I think there was one uveitis or iritis case; but macular edema, as I recall, was found in 14 to 20%. Sixty-two percent of those resolved, leaving unresolved macular edema in 7%. There was no instance of phthisis bulbi, and retinal detachments occurred in only 5% or five patients out of 103. One of those cases detached two years later, and another one detached one year after surgery.

Jaffe That really answers it because you have the facts.

· · ·

Question   Dr. Jaffe, what is your experience with cocaine drops and osmotic
agents to relieve vitreous touch?

Jaffe   I haven't been as successful as Marvin Sears in relieving vitreous touch
or pupillary block with the use of cocaine. As a matter of fact, I've never
been successful with this particular procedure. I'm sure there are others
that have, and I think Dr. Norton always makes this point. Never argue with
another fellow who has seen something. Probably at that time he saw a
good result from this. The only point I'd like to make is that our journals are
full of observations we make. We have an Archives, an AJO, et cetera; but
there's a bigger journal that is so much fuller than these journals and it's
called "The Journal of I Take It All Back."

It's unfortunate how often we get into a journal with a very preliminary
observation; and you know, with the use of cocaine, it's not so bad because I
don't think eyeballs have been knocked out by cocaine. I'm sorry for this veer-
ing away from your question, but I've had no success with the treatment.

McClure   What about the use of cryo for vitreous touch? Is your answer the
same?

Jaffe   Well, if you remember, just before John McClean died there was an
editorial in the Archives "Cryo—See or No." Drysdale and Shea after a single
experience of vitreal-corneal adherence reported cryo as a treatment. John
McClean tried this on one of his cases and produced a total decompensation
of the cornea. The rationale was that you temporarily destroy the endothelium
and thereby allow the vitreous to separate from the cornea, and then hopefully
a regeneration of endothelium occurs while the vitreous has found its way
back to the level of the iris. I think that falls in the category again of "I take
it all back." I'd never recommend this as a treatment since there are so many
more effective ways of accomplishing it which are less damaging.

• • •

McClure   Are there any other opinions on the panel?

Ryan   Just certainly to agree with what Dr. Jaffe has said. Namely, we have
tried cocaine without success and again haven't tried freezing. It would seem
to me that, technique-wise, the question is really going to come down to
what are the indications and how to intervene, and certainly Dr. Jaffe has
emphasized this in his talk. Namely, there are a number of different variables
that one has to deal with. We've evolved into a rationale where the individual
must show progression of the area of corneal decompensation.

Now, again, once you get to that stage, you're up against the problem of
how do you know before it goes too far. In one case that I've seen that
progressed from 3½ to 4 mm of corneal vitreal adhesion, a Los Angeles
surgeon intervened through the pars plana, and the individual subsequently
cleared the entire central cornea. Although this is only an isolated case, I'm
illustrating this as an approach; I'm not saying it's the final answer. We think

the preferred technique for removing vitreous in the most atraumatic fashion is through a pars plana vitrectomy.

Jaffe   We've had a few successes with corneal touch just as you described, Steve, at Bascom Palmer with vitrectomy. As I said earlier, that may be the best way to go and it may be better than the Leahey treatment because you actually get rid of the vitreous rather than just pushing it back. The only way we're going to find out is by enough cases being accumulated so that we can get enough facts. These facts have to be repeated in enough people's hands.

Douvas   I can add a series of five cases of corneal decompensation and vitreous touch I approached through a healthy limbal incision to accomplish the same thing, rather than through the pars plana, with good results.

Ryan   Just purely from the technical point of view, one of the factors one encounters is where the cornea is decompensated despite going through all your maneuvers to try and clear the cornea, you are going to be left with stromal edema. In point of fact, that is a big advantage to have the clear area, especially in cases like this, so you can amputate the vitreous around that area and then go back with vitrectomy.

Douvas   I might add though that frequently there's vitreous incarcerated into the wound. The question there is when I approach it through the limbus, I've tried to hook these strands with an extremely fine Bond iris hook rather than a spatula that would slip off. Of course, it may suffice to cut these strands off posteriorly if you can; but frequently they are so adherent to the iris that they persist even though you've done a clear vitrectomy.

Peyman   I'd also like to emphasize one fact, and that is, when to do this procedure. I had experience in two cases of vitreous touch and corneal decompensation. After vitrectomy through pars plana, the visual acuity improved; but there was persistent corneal edema, and it hasn't gone away yet. I think if the corneal endothelium is damaged enough then you'll have persistent corneal edema even if you improve the vision. If I wanted to choose a procedure I'd use, as Dr. Ryan suggested, it would be the pars plana approach rather than the anterior approach.

Ryan   I have a mild disagreement with Dr. Douvas. Although I prefer a limbal approach to mainly anterior problems, the reason I prefer a pars plana approach in vitreous touch is that it's easier to perform a more complete vitrectomy by this route than through the limbal incision. By going through the pars plana, one is able, after working in the anterior chamber, to go posteriorly and do more of a vitrectomy with good visualization. Going through the limbus, the problem is parallax. If the eye later comes to penetrating keratoplasty, at least I feel I'll have done a good enough vitrectomy to make the keratoplasty easier as a subsequent procedure.

• • •

Jaffe   Could I ask Dr. Coleman a question? I was so impressed with what you did that I think they're going to start to call you Buck. You're the Buck

Rogers of this generation of what we're doing. I thought it was fantastic. I'd like to ask you something that's much more minor than that. What is the finest resolution you can get along the ultrasonic axial length of the globe?

Coleman   The original equipment we designed was specifically to do that. I was originally interested in disproving the Helmholtz theory of accommodation about six years ago. I tried to get as accurate a measurement as we could using ultrasound. We really can make a measurement technically to 30 μ of tissue thickness, based on calculations on metal blocks and knowing the velocity of sound. Sound velocities do vary in an eye with a cataract. I assume you're asking the question for measurement of intraocular lenses. The problem is this: when we measure the axial length of an eye with a cataract, the velocity of sound in the cataract varies from roughly 1,629 to 1,670 meters per second. That variation in sound velocity will mean that our total measurement will be inaccurate to a variable amount, perhaps by as much as 0.1 mm.

Jaffe   If it's just 0.1 mm, I'd be very happy. It's a practical point if that is the resolution you'd expect to achieve by teaching technicians to do this kind of work with currently available equipment.

Coleman   Yes. Well, if one uses a 20 megahertz transducer, the problems that one has are really three: (1) you have to use a high-frequency transducer with a very narrow beam; (2) you can't deform the globe; and (3) the standoff probe called for is inaccurate. The beam must be narrow so that it isn't striking the edge of the back of the eye but rather is right at the point of the macula. You cannot deform the globe in any way. So, if the technician is making the measurement, he needs to have a standoff probe that just barely touches the cornea and doesn't press on it and doesn't deform it. This is the main inaccuracy in most ultrasound systems. They use the contact probe directly on the cornea with no standoffs, i.e., waterbath, so the main bang of the transducer is lost in the anterior corneal echo. Overall, I think we can get to within less than one quarter of a diopter with the understanding that the velocities of sound variations will throw sound off just a little bit.

·   ·   ·

Cockerham   This question is to the panel, regarding two patients, one from the audience and one from a case I saw recently. Both were young male adults, one of whom went to the bathroom and another was involved in a bout of sneezing, and both developed preretinal hemorrhages. What causes it, what is the course, and what do you do for it? Do you see those cases occasionally?

Okun   I don't know what the cause is. I've seen it and you can conjecture as to the cause—a tremendous Valsalva effect probably—a tremendous increase of venous pressure and a blowout from some place. Usually it is a young kid performing some type of calisthenics, a tremendous sneeze, or something of that nature. They usually clear quite well. I think I've seen three, and they have all cleared quite well.

The disappointing thing is that I can't find a darned thing after they have cleared. I'm looking for a little spot of neovascularization or something that might explain it and never find it. I would liken it to what happens with a subretinal hemorrhage. Boom—you get a hemorrhage. The next thing you know, both eyes have preretinal hemorrhages and then maybe even vitreous hemorrhages. Of course, they usually don't clear. You examine those eyes in the laboratory postmortem and you still can't be 100% sure where the hemorrhage is coming from, but probably from some of the larger veins or some of the weaker-walled vessels.

Cockerham   Do you find any blood abnormalities or any vascular disease?

Okun   I honestly haven't looked. They seem like all healthy people and they've all done quite well afterwards.

Gitter   I haven't seen the type of patient you describe, Walter; but I have seen what I know all of us have seen occasionally, and that is macular or para-macular spontaneous hemorrhages in young people who have no obvious reason for macular hemorrhage and who, when completely worked up—including fluorescein angiography and everything else—have no detectable abnormalities. When followed, these intraretinal and occasionally preretinal hemorrhages clear without sequela.

Dr. Andrew Hubbard recently studied a series of four or five (I must now have about nine) of these patients ranging in age from 18 to 40 with no significant history. They complain of some blurring of vision, usually 20/30 to 20/40; and over a period of 1 to 2 months, the hemorrhage goes away. Maybe this is just minor manifestation of the more major preretinal hemor-rhage described by Dr. Okun, and perhaps they are due to increase in venous pressure, I don't know.

Douvas   I might just make a comment that as a resident at Iowa, we had one fellow who came into the clinic, I think, on three different occasions. He prac-ticed yoga and stood on his head for 20 minutes, and on at least two of the occasions I saw him with his retina full of hemorrhages. As I recall now, those were intraretinal hemorrhages, but this was the result of his yoga and we tried to discourage him from continuing but he refused.

· · ·

McClure   Concerning vitreous loss at the time of cataract surgery, I would like to poll the panel as to who is using the newer forms of vitrectomy instru-ments versus the Weck sponge anterior vitrectomy, and what are the advan-tages and disadvantages of each?

Douvas   Obviously I'm using the Roto-Extractor in the management of this. To me, the advantage is I'm able to pull up my sutures, which have been preplaced prior to lens delivery, and then insert the instrument through one suture that is left loose and do the vitrectomy under a controlled situation wherein the globe is being constantly pressurized with infusion as the vitreous is being removed. When we are satisfied that we have cleared the anterior and posterior chambers of vitreous, and going no deeper with the instrument than what would normally be the plane of the posterior lens capsule, we remove the instrument and insert Miochol into the eye. We see if the pupil constricts down and look for the slightest suggestion of any pupillary tinting or notching. Then, if we see any, we slip an iris hook into the opposite pole, a very fine (Bond) iris hook, and hook this strand from the wound where it may be incarcerated, to free it.

Coleman   I think there's a practical matter in having the vitrectomy instrument readily available at the time of routine intracapsular extraction where vitreous loss really isn't expected. I'm still waiting for a case in which I could do that. I've been looking for one. In addition, it would take too long in our setup to get the instrument ready because we don't have it ready and on hand. Another thing, if you're doing intracapsular extraction, you have a big open wound.

Douvas   In my case, the instrument is set up, it's sterile. We pull up our sutures, and time is not a factor there. Unfortunately I had my only expulsive hemorrhage trying the Weck sponge technique. It may have happened anyway. Maybe I didn't quit soon enough. I don't know. In other words, I depressurized the eye in an elderly patient with brittle vessels, and he let loose on me. At least we didn't lose the globe, but I didn't restore his vision.

Ryan   I would tend to second what Dr. Coleman said as far as the practical problem of setting up the vitrectomy unit, and again I'm not really concerned about our schedules but rather just the time the patient is on the table. I think again that, if it's the type of an eye where one can do a satisfactory Kasner anterior vitrectomy, that would seem to work quite well. On the other hand, there are those patients that—if you don't have a ring on, if this is something that isn't anticipated and you get into the problem of that tremendous scleral collapse—then to do the adequate vitrectomy that might be indicated, you may have to use the Roto-Extractor.

Jaffe   I have no experience with any of the vitrectomy machines, but I'm just wondering. Maybe we should look into Kaufmann's little vitrector. It's so little, easily available, sterile, and could be used at a moment's notice. Maybe this would be better, I don't know.

Ryan   You'd be the one to really decide that. I think that in my own mind my preconceived notion is that you feel the vitreous is continuing to come from choroid expanding. There's no question that you want to get that globe closed quickly. I'd agree to use the Concept device. In general, where it is a vitreous loss without any evidence of continuing pressure from the back, don't you feel that the open sky is perfectly adequate?

Jaffe   I only feel that way on the basis of the fact that this is what I've been doing, but I really haven't compared it with other methods. I was thinking while Nick was talking about his case that the eye was open too long and you had an expulsive hemorrhage. This is one of the factors. It's awfully nice to be able to get in and out with that. I think David Kasner would like it. I think we would irritate the iris a little unless, as you stated before . . . I don't know. You certainly will leave less sponge in the eye.

Kasner   One of the reasons Dr. Machemer developed his machine was because putting a sponge in and out of the pupil irritated the iris, which created the uveitis and general inflammation postoperatively in the open sky technique. He thought that—if you could just avoid touching the iris, stick the tube in, and do the vitrectomy that way—it would be less inflammatory; and it's true. If you don't touch the iris, you get less postoperative inflammation, which is why I don't use the spear sponges when I go down through the pupil. I chop up the Weck sponges until they are 1 × 5 mm, little slivers, to go through the pupil.

I had a 750-dollar vitrector made up for me with a battery and a 0.4 mm tip just to do this thing that the vitrector is designed to do. I stuck it through the pupil when I had a vitreous loss; and watching that thing go so slowly trying to eat up the vitreous, I put it down and picked up the sponges, which could take out large globs in a short period of time. The opening I used on the vitrector that I designed was 0.4 mm. The commercially available unit (Concept) is about 0.9 mm or 1 mm or 0.8 mm. It makes a difference. If the opening is big that little gadget may be good if it can take out the vitreous fast, because if you don't rub the iris the postoperative complications are less.

Okun   I might comment that there is a lot to be said for high-speed cutting, and that is you get multiple fine tissue slices; you don't get long spaghetti pulls. So at a high speed (say 1,000 rpm) you get a lot of fast slices; and in terms of speed again, it's a question of what your duty cycle is: whether it's an instrument with a short duty cycle, mainly closed two thirds of the time, as it is in the instruments designed with a hole opposite a hole, or one that might be open half the time with a high-speed cutting.

Peyman   My experience is limited to penetrating keratoplasty and vitrectomy. In that regard, with my instrument, at the time I was doing penetrating keratoplasty and wanted to do combined vitrectomy before we had the instrument, I was also using the Weck sponges; but now, with my instrument, it doesn't take more than 4 or 5 minutes to remove practically the whole anterior vitreous without any problem.

•   •   •

Cockerham   I'd like to ask Dr. Jaffe two questions and make a couple of comments. First, which lens do you prefer, the Hruby lens or the Goldmann posterior pole lens? I personally feel that the Goldmann lens is vastly superior in doing just about anything. Also I wonder if in your examination you've used the horizontal slit and utilized the ascension phenomenon. I've been impressed at how a lot of what you think will be adhesions really are only apparent; and when you set the vitreous in motion, you see a smooth posterior hyaloid face move out from the retina and get the feeling that there really isn't an adhesion. I just wondered how you approach this.

Jaffe   I more or less agree with you. I think a Hruby lens, as Dr. Douvas used to say, is a Mickey Mouse thing compared to using a good three-mirror lens. I very much like to use the Thorpe four-mirror, which I find easy to use. I've also adapted on my Zeiss slit lamp the horizontal angle lamp, which I can turn to any angle I like. I purposely got it for the reason you described.

The ascension phenomenon is a fantastic thing to look for, because it even gives you a prognostic significance on vitreous hemorrhages and endophthalmitis. In others words, when I see these membranes jump up and down, I feel a little better than during ascension; they go staccato or don't move at all. I like to use that as a prognostic sign. I think the horizontal view you described today is extremely useful.

•   •   •

Cockerham   Dr. Shields, what are your indications for vitreous biopsy, and tell a little bit about the technique.

Shields   I'd like to say a few points about what we think are possible indications. I haven't had much experience with the technique. Maybe Dr. Federman can comment on the technique with the instruments that we've used at our institution.

One main indication that is really getting a lot of attention recently is the concept of reticulum cell sarcoma. This is very interesting, because any number of people realize that if you have a patient with the onset of uveitis in middle age or older age you may suspect this diagnosis; and there are instances where the only apparent involvement in the body is in the eye. It can be an infiltration of the retina or the choroid, and in a few cases now there've just been cells in the vitreous. In these cases there've been a number of well-documented cases where they have gone in and made the diagnosis. And then, of course, there're the therapeutic implications, that we won't get into. This is one indication.

There may be another indication—an occasional case of retinoblastoma. If you have a child with an unexplained inflamed eye, and you don't know what's going on, and you think it may be a severe uveitis or endophthalmitis from some unknown cause—you can go in and sometimes demonstrate retinoblastoma cells.

In my experience these are two things that we've diagnosed in our institution with this technique. Also, another point is that if you suspect one of these things and you only find benign inflammatory cells, then you can rule out a tumor or something severe like that.

Okun   I'd just like to caution those of you who think you may want to make the diagnosis of retinoblastoma or malignant melanoma through a pars plana incision. I'm very much concerned that there could be leakage around the sclerotomy site. It's been reported that the diagnosis of retinoblastoma has been made through an anterior chamber tap, which I think would be much clearer and cleaner. As far as malignant melanoma is concerned, I think we'd be better off using techniques already available. We have quite a few, and I'd guess that we could diagnose 99% of those with what we have.

8

Vitrectomy instrumentation, Roto-Extractor indications, and techniques and results

NICHOLAS G. DOUVAS

This chapter is subdivided into sections dealing with instrumentation (design and requirements), the Douvas Roto-Extractor, and results and analysis of 100 consecutive Roto-Extractor cases.

INSTRUMENTATION
Design

There are three cutting principles employed in vitrectomy instruments: the grinding shear, the circular scissors, and the guillotine.

In instruments utilizing the *grinding shear* cutting principle, an axial thrust pushes the rotating male cone against the fixed female component. One version has a fixed hole matching a rotating hole. The grinding shear must of necessity work slowly. The instrument has a short duty cycle because the aspiration port is closed about two thirds of the time. Another version incorporates an auger that also works with a spring-loaded axial thrust to effect the grinding shear. The difference is that with this auger principle there is a continuous feed since the cutter opening is never fully closed. Therefore the instrument does not cut fully free at any time unless there is backflushing.

In instruments utilizing the *circular scissors* cutting principle, as exemplified by the Roto-Extractor, the vitrectomy tips are of a triple-walled construction. The double-edged cutter blade is flared not only posteriorly but to the side to create a spring form that provides scissorlike contact with the inner cutting aperture edges. The blade may be rotated up to 1,000 rpm in a continuous direction, or it may be oscillated without making more than a 360° turn in either direction.

In instruments utilizing the *guillotine* cutting principle, the blade rotates axially, cutting either internally or externally.

Requirements
Mandatory requirements

All instruments must provide adequate infusion without a jetstream force. There must be adequate vacuum, controlled by one means or another. The surgeon should be in full command of cutting at all times, preferably by foot control.

Mandatory vitrectomy instrument requirements include the ability to aspirate without cutting and to cut without aspirating. I believe this is very important. (Other authors may not agree.) It is equally important to be able to cut without aspiration as to be able to cut with aspiration. Many times the surgeon needs to cut totally free of tissue at the aspiration port. Some of the continuous-feed instruments lack this ability.

Desirable features

Desirable vitrectomy instrument features include a means to prevent internal liquid or vacuum short-circuiting between the infusion port and the aspiration port. This requires triple-walled probe construction.

There should be an optional oscillatory double-cutting edge feature, at least for the rotary type of instrument.

There should be no exposed moving parts within the infusion port. The probe tips should be interchangeable and of the same diameter, and there should be the ability to vary cutting aperture openings because of tissue bridging effects.

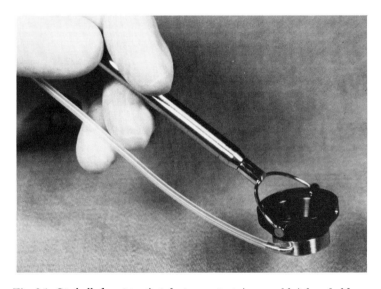

Fig. 8-1. Gimballed assistant's infusion contact (removable) lens holder.

Tissue character varies; some tissue can be impacted in a small opening whereas other tissue is best impacted in a larger opening.

There should be the ability to vary the cutting speed and vacuum pull to sustain a given minimal vacuum without circulating nurse assistance. There should be minimal interruption of suction during cutting so the tissue (i.e., the luxated lens material) will not be lost when the cutter is activated. There should be high-speed cutting for small-tissue slicing and to avoid spaghetti-like tissue cuttings that cause instrument clogging.

There should be a fiber-optic light pipe or sleeve, a trocar and cannula, and an infusion contact lens with an optional gimballed assistant's handle (Fig. 8-1) for use when the surgeon has both hands occupied with two instruments in the eye.

The rack-and-pinion syringe drive of Charles (Fig. 8-2) has distinct advantages, such as one-hand aspiration. Manual aspiration with proprioceptive feedback to a competent assistant, however, will never be exceeded by any automated instrument because the human mind is a computer that is tough to beat (Fig. 8-3). All the same, if an automated system is employed, it must attempt to provide equal control and information to the surgeon while he maintains his eyes at the microscope without turning around to look at the dials.

Undesirable features

Although other men may disagree, the following are my ideas on the subject of undesirable features of vitrectomy instruments:

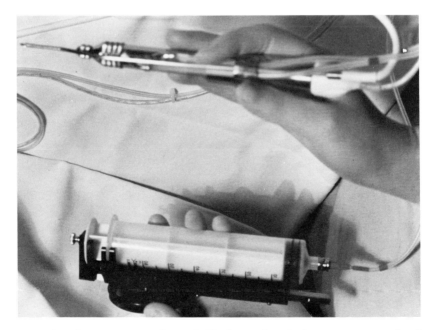

Fig. 8-2. Rack-and-pinion syringe drive of Charles used with the Roto-Extractor handpiece.

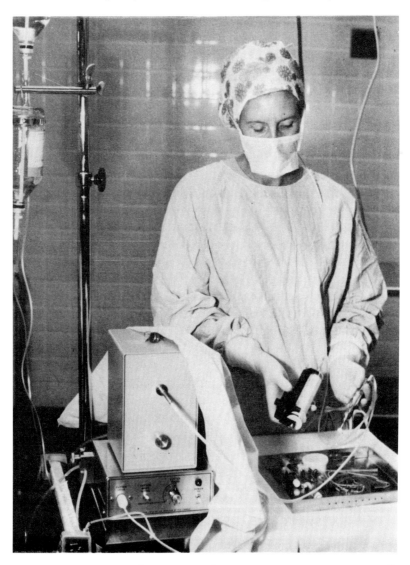

Fig. 8-3. Roto-Extractor surgical assistant with instrument system components (foot pedal not shown).

Instruments which are unable to aspirate without simultaneous cutting are undesirable. There are many times when aspiration alone is highly desirable.

Finger control of suction or cutting is also undesirable. After prolonged surgery there is a loss of finger agility that precludes delicate maneuvering close to the retina. Probe tip rotation of 180° or more necessitates an awkward hand position with finger-controlled instruments. A rotating finger control may be of some benefit; but if rotation with a light pipe is indicated, this also will be awkward. Furthermore, a pressure gradient may exist when the finger is off the vacuum hole. If the eye is pressurized above atmospheric pressure, fluid and

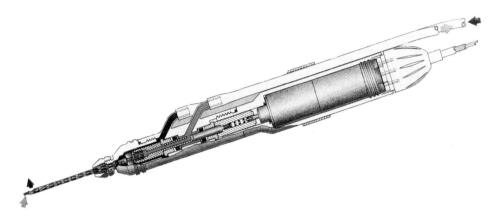

Fig. 8-4. Roto-Extractor handpiece flow diagram with motor cartridge, cutter set, cable, and tubing.

tissue material will be forced into the cutter opening, with inadvertent tissue incarceration.

A 0.6 mm external pistonlike movement at the end of a reciprocating guillotine-like instrument is undesirable since it precludes working close to the retina.

The continuous auger feed principle with uninterrupted aspiration is undesirable because it prevents cutting totally free of tissue and results in tissue incarceration into the instrument. Consequently backflushing and reverse cutting are required to cut free of tissue. The backflush ability exists in only one of the two instruments incorporating this auger principle.

Distant and separate fiber-optic light probe systems may result in visibility that is inadequate at the end of the cutting probe because of difficulty in aligning the fiber-optic light in a heavily organized eye.

Distant and separate sclerotomy for an infusion cannula may lead to instrument clogging because of inadequate available infused vehicular fluid in a heavily organized eye necessary to carry tissue cuttings through the aspiration passages.

DOUVAS ROTO-EXTRACTOR

The Roto-Extractor cross section is illustrated in Fig. 8-4. The instrument's handpiece with its light pipe is seen in Fig. 8-5.

The Roto-Extractor comes equipped with interchangeable probe tips (Fig. 8-6) of both end-core cutting and side cutting design. The trephine end-core cutter may be used for preliminary phacofragmentation and hydrolysis. The side-cutting design offers two sizes—0.6 mm and 0.4 mm. The 0.4 mm size can be stopped in a half-closed position and effectively narrowed to a 0.2 mm opening when necessary to impact a thin strand that otherwise could not be impacted because of fluid seepage around the edges of the larger cutting aperture.

The fiber-optic light pipe assembly is shown in Fig. 8-7.

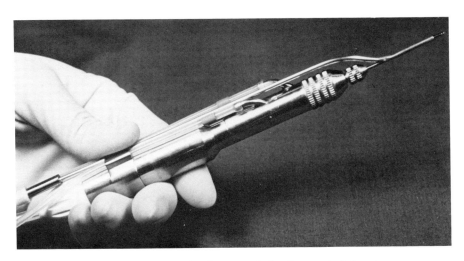

Fig. 8-5. Roto-Extractor handpiece with the fiber-optic light pipe.

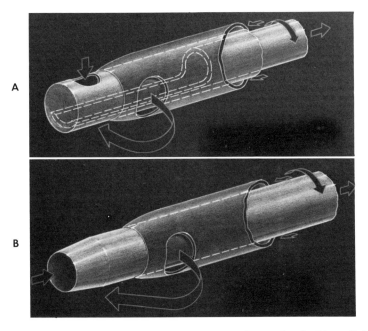

Fig. 8-6. Diagram of, **A,** the triple-walled side cutter and, **B,** the double-walled trephine end-core cutter.

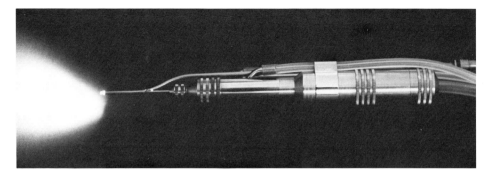

Fig. 8-7. Roto-Extractor fiber-optic illumination.

A high-speed clockwise or optional clockwise/counterclockwise oscillatory double-cutting edge rotation is of value. The continuous single-direction mode is faster, smoother, and generally most effective when used with the trephine end-core cutter for initial lens fragmentation and honeycombing. It permits a faster vitrectomy when there is little resistance to cutting, and it promotes longer motor life. The oscillatory cutting action is safer when removing iris, which otherwise may have a propensity to become wrapped in case of cutter malfunction; it frequently permits more effective cutting of a taut anterior lens capsule that tends to slide off a cutter moving in a single direction.

The 0.4 mm protected side cutter is usually more effective than the 0.6 or 0.8 mm probe tip because of bridging or saddle phenomena. Every tissue has a different characteristic—and one size of cutter works better in one case, and another in another.

Taut vitreous bands are often effectively cut with the oscillatory mode when little progress is being made with single-direction cutting. The oscillatory mode is not effective with the trephine end-core cutter for lens fragmentation because it tends to cause a firm lens to rock back and forth. Sometimes in using the oscillatory mode while impacting dense postcataract lens membrane, the surgeon encounters a rocking effect that prevents full impaction and cutting at full speed; but after slowing the motor to two-thirds cutter speed, he is able to make progress because of the increased capability to impact tissue more deeply in the instrument.

The advantage of the triple-tubed cutters has already been alluded to (i.e., the prevention of internal liquid or vacuum short-circuiting so that vacuum efficiency at the aspiration port is increased to better impact cataractous material or vitreous for cutting and aspiration). A vacuum pull across a two-tube bearing seal cannot occur to impact vitreous or cataract into the infusion port, where it can be wrapped or caught on an exposed rotating or oscillating type of shaft.

In a two-tube system, obviously, the bearing seal between infusion and aspiration chambers has to be less than perfect; otherwise, the moving element cannot move. As long as a two-tube instrument is new and fits well, this ap-

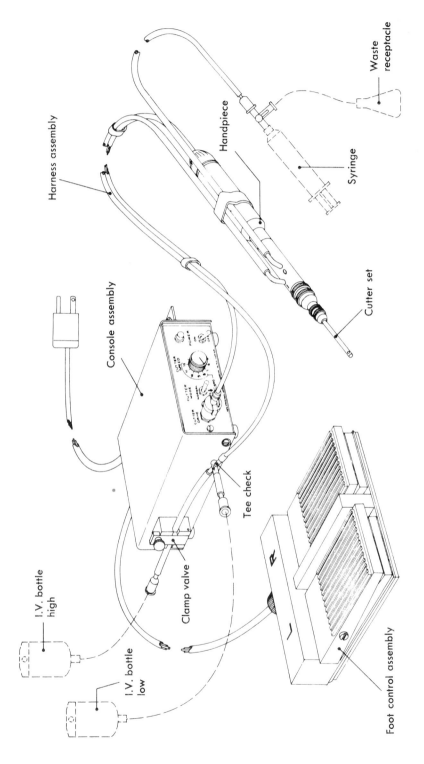

Fig. 8-8. Roto-Extractor system component arrangement.

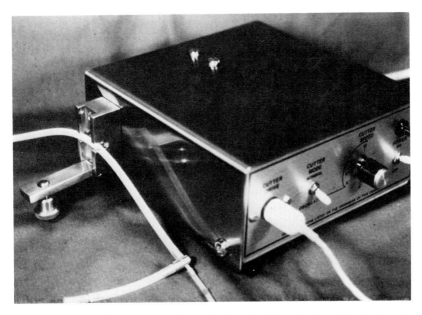

Fig. 8-9. Roto-Extractor electronic console with a T check for the low infusion bottle and a solenoid clamp for the high infusion bottle.

parently is not much of a problem; but with wear, a number of problems can develop. The increased intraocular pressure resulting from contact lens manipulation during vitrectomy may force vitreous into the infusion port, where it may be caught on an exposed moving element in a two-tube system.

The system component arrangement of the Roto-Extractor (Fig. 8-8) consists of two infusion bottles, a control console, a handpiece with manual aspiration, and a dual foot pedal. The left side of the pedal permits cutting only. A sequential pedal on the right side initially activates the solenoid that opens the higher infusion bottle to permit greater flow. Further right pedal depression activates cutting.

The console and tubing (with a T check to the low infusion bottle and a solenoid clamp to the high infusion bottle) are seen in Fig. 8-9. There are a speed-control knob and a cutter-mode switch for either continuous single-direction cutting or an oscillatory clockwise/counterclockwise cutting. An off-on switch is also present on the console front panel.

The instrument is housed in a sterilizing box with the various cutting tips and two wrenches for cutter-tip changing and spindle-body servicing when needed. The fiber-optic light pipe is positioned along the periphery of the box, and an infusion Goldmann contact lens is contained in a small white case (Fig. 8-10).

The Roto-Extractor may be gas sterilized on a cold cycle or flash autoclaved for successive procedures if the motor cartridge and the white case containing the Goldmann contact lens are removed from the sterilizing box. Although the fiber-optic light pipe may be autoclaved, it has a longer useful life when gas

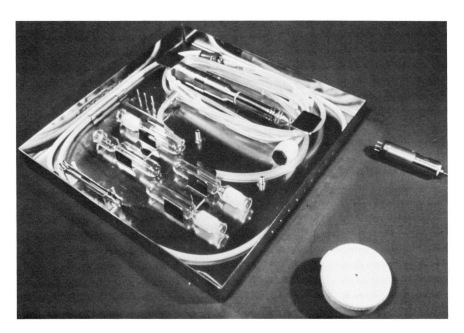

Fig. 8-10. Roto-Extractor sterilizing box with the contact lens container and motor cartridge removed for flash autoclaving.

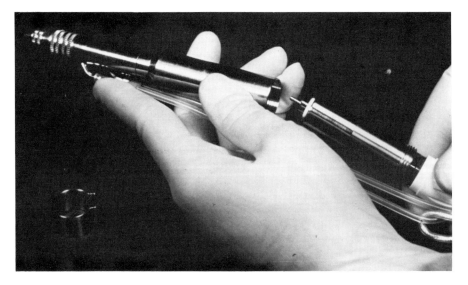

Fig. 8-11. Insertion of the motor cartridge into the Roto-Extractor handpiece motor housing.

or cold-solution sterilized. The contact lens may be cold-solution sterilized, but the tubing had best be autoclaved. The motor does not have to be sterilized if care is taken with its insertion into the motor housing (Fig. 8-11).

If the motor was gas sterilized for the first procedure, its sterility can be maintained with proper technique between successive operations while the sterilizing box and contents are flash autoclaved.

Table 8-1. Roto-Extractor operations (100 cases)

	Procedure/Approach	*Cases*
Congenital and developmental cataracts		12
Primary surgery	Lim (4)	
	PP (5)	
Previous surgery with postcataract membrane	Lim (3)	
Traumatic cataract		17
Primary surgery	Lim (7)	
Previous surgery with postcataract membrane	Lim (10)	
Cataracta complicata secondary to uveitis	Lim (1)	3
	PP (2)	
Massive anterior chamber hyphema with glaucoma		2
Complications of intracapsular cataract extraction		19
Bullous keratitis with vitreous touch	(5)	
Updrawn pupil after vitreous loss	(3)	
Miotic pupil with cloudy vitreous	(1)	
Iris–ciliary body implantation cyst with vitreous adherence	(1)	
Postcataract membrane	(2)	
Pupillary block glaucoma	(1)	
Totally luxated lens with phacolytic glaucoma	(2)	
Subluxated senile cataract with vitreous herniated into anterior chamber	(1)	
Iris–ciliary body implantation cyst with vitreous adherence	(2)	
Aphakic glaucoma filtering operation with vitreous present in filtration area	(1)	
Complications of phacoemulsification		2
Vitreous in anterior chamber	(1)	
Opaque postcataract membrane	(1)	
Persistent hyperplastic primary vitreous		1
Traumatic massive vitreous hemorrhage		5
Contusion	V (PP) (1)	
	L&V (PP) (1)	
Perforating	L&V (PP) (3)	
Vitreous opacification and retinal detachment secondary to uveitis	L&V (PP) (1)	2
	V (PP) (1)	
Massive unabsorbed vitreous hemorrhage secondary to branch vein occlusion	L&V (PP) (1)	2
	V (PP) (1)	
Massive unabsorbed vitreous hemorrhage secondary to hypertension	V (PP)	1
Diabetic vitreous hemorrhage, unabsorbed	V (PP)	10
Diabetic vitreous hemorrhage and cataract	L&V (PP)	24

     Code: Lim, Limbal incision
             PP, Pars plana incision
             L, Lensectomy
             V, Vitrectomy

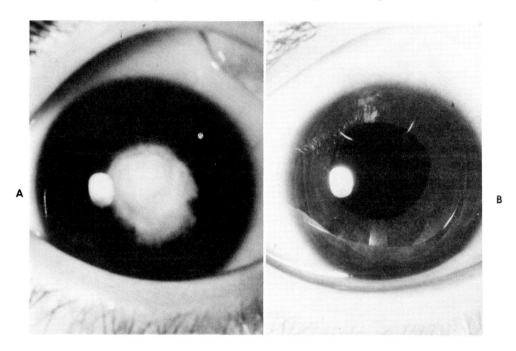

Fig. 8-12. Congenital cataract. **A,** Preoperative; **B,** postoperative appearance.

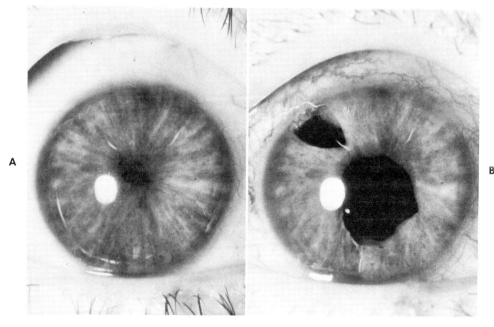

Fig. 8-13. **A,** Previously operated on (twice) congenital cataract. **B,** Postoperative appearance after use of the Roto-Extractor.

INDICATIONS AND RESULTS OF 100 CONSECUTIVE
ROTO-EXTRACTOR OPERATIONS

Table 8-1 outlines 100 consecutive Roto-Extractor operations and provides an idea as to indications and results of these 100 cases, which are subdivided into thirteen categories.

There were twelve cases of congenital or developmental cataract done by either a limbal incision or a pars plana approach. Pre- and postoperative photographs of an example of congenital cataract are shown in Fig. 8-12. There were also patients who had had previous surgery and were approached by a limbal incision. Fig. 8-13 illustrates one of these patients, who had had two previous operations before being improved from 20/70 to 20/20. Much of the lensectomy was accomplished through a peripheral iridectomy.

In doing a lensectomy on developmental cataracts, the surgeon enters the capsular bag by drilling into it with the trephine end-core cutter. He then makes multiple probe thrusts within the capsular bag with backflushing (by the assistant through the aspiration chamber) to hydrate the lens while the high-speed continuous rotary cutter is used. This fragmentation and hydration of the lens may persist for 5 minutes or more to soften and mature the lens prior to aspiration, which is performed within the capsular bag so the operator does not have to chase lens material all around the anterior chamber. The posterior capsule is carefully avoided to obviate posterior luxation of lens material. After lens fragmentation, aspiration is started and only what comes easily is taken with the trephine prior to switching to a side cutter.

A total of seventeen cases of traumatic cataract underwent Roto-Extractor lensectomy. All seventeen were performed via the limbal incision. Fig. 8-14 illustrates the pre- and postoperative appearance 9 days after surgery of a 28-year-old eye. Cases with previous surgery and dense postsurgical cataracts were also operated, as shown in Fig. 8-15.

Cataracta complicata secondary to uveitis totalled three cases. Fig. 8-16 illustrates what proved to be a very dense cataracta complicata, which was removed almost entirely in the capsular bag without posterior lens luxation. The procedure was lengthy and tedious. A pars plana approach was utilized because of previously known vitreous uveitic opacification.

There were two cases of traumatic anterior chamber hyphema with secondary glaucoma. Fig. 8-17 shows the postoperative appearance of one of these eyes, which still has bloodstaining of the cornea inferiorly. No lens opacities developed.

There were nineteen cases with complications following cataract extraction.

Fig. 8-18 is of an aphakic one-eyed patient whose presenting complaint was of flashes and floaters. This patient's other eye had been lost because of a totally detached retina. She was under treatment with echothiophate iodide. She had a miotic tented pupil that would not dilate. A murky horsetailed vitreous herniated through the miotic pupil and precluded visualization of her retina. Although initial visual acuity after cataract surgery was 20/25, vision subsequently became 20/200 with increasing opacification of the horsetailed vitreous.

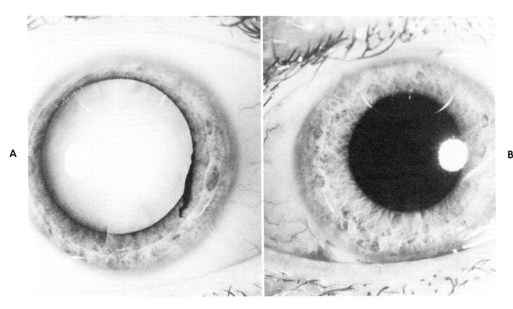

Fig. 8-14. Traumatic cataract in a 28-year-old patient. **A,** Preoperative; **B,** postoperative (ninth day) appearance.

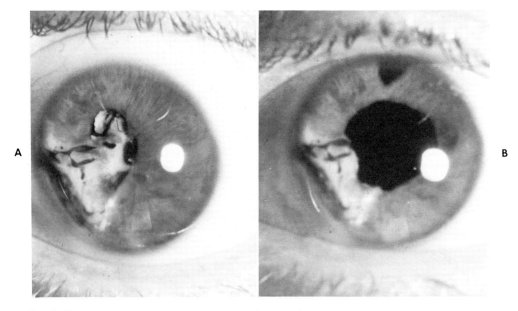

Fig. 8-15. Dense traumatic postcataract membrane. **A,** Preoperative; **B,** postoperative appearance.

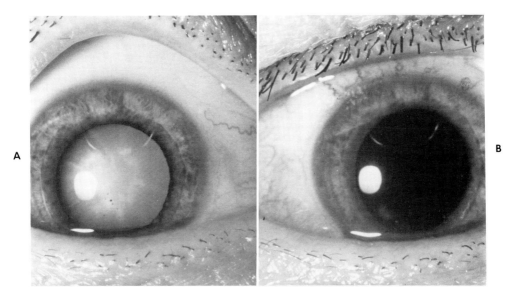

Fig. 8-16. Dense cataracta complicata secondary to uveitis. **A,** Preoperative; **B,** postoperative appearance.

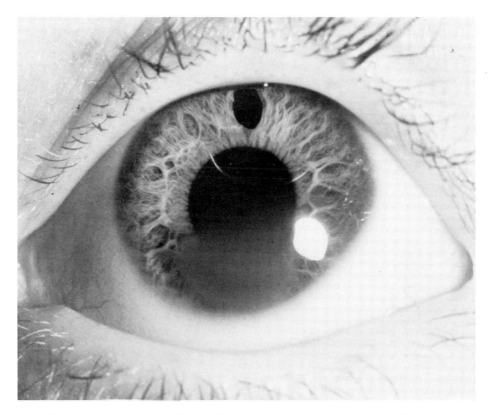

Fig. 8-17. Anterior chamber hyphema with secondary glaucoma. Postoperative appearance with residual corneal bloodstaining.

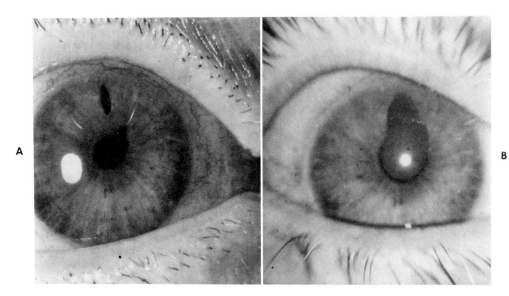

Fig. 8-18. Aphakic glaucoma with miotic pupil filled with mushroomed opacified horsetailed vitreous. **A,** Preoperative tented pupil; **B,** postoperative clear red reflex with sector iridectomy.

The surgical plan was to remove the murky vitreous and enlarge the pupillary opening by performing an iridectomy via a limbal incision. The anterior chamber angle was first swept with a fine iris hook and a vitreous strand was caught and pulled from the wound. The anterior chamber was then reentered with the Roto-Extractor (0.4 mm side cutter), which was briefly pulsed in an oscillatory mode to create a sector iridectomy. An anterior microsurgical vitrectomy was also performed. The retina was found attached. Visual acuity improved to 20/25 within a week. Because a relative vitreal pupillary block had been eliminated by the shallow anterior vitrectomy, no subsequent glaucoma therapy was required.

Fig. 8-19 shows an updrawn pupil in a 28-year-old aphakic eye that was complicated by massive unabsorbed vitreous hemorrhage and vitreous incarceration into the wound. A pars plana vitrectomy and iridectomy were performed, with good visual result.

The correct manner of performing an iridectomy with the Roto-Extractor is as follows:

1. The assistant impacts the iris tissue into the cutter opening by aspiration to create a "morning glory" effect with only minimum vacuum necessary to hold onto the iris.
2. The surgeon pulses the cutter in an oscillatory mode for a single cut of iris.
3. There should be no residual vacuum pull on the iris, nor should there be peripheral iris tug or any tendency to wrapping or pulling that might create a dialysis.

With senile cataracts the limitation of a combined lensectomy-vitrectomy is a grade II nuclear sclerosis. If harder (III or IV) lenses are attempted, a two-instrument lens-crushing technique may become necessary. The Roto-Extractor is not

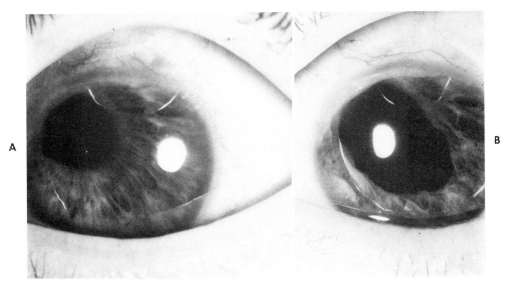

Fig. 8-19. Aphakic updrawn pupil after vitreous loss. **A,** Preoperative; **B,** postoperative appearance.

recommended for senile cataract extraction unless vitrectomy is the main indication.

Fig. 8-20 illustrates a post-phacoemulsification complication and the post-Roto-Extractor result. This patient had undergone phacoemulsification elsewhere, with vitreous loss that required conversion and vitrectomy by the Weck sponge technique. A postcataract membrane persisted with a small central opening. The periphery of the membrane, however, was opaque and thus precluded adequate visualization of an underlying bullous retinal detachment. The Roto-Extractor was employed prior to surgical repair of the detachment.

There was one case of PHPV (Fig. 8-21) in which an inadvertent sector iridectomy was created. This complication can occur readily with uncontrolled cutting and suction while working close to the iris.

Five of the 100 consecutive Roto-Extractor procedures were for traumatic vitreous hemorrhage. Two resulted from contusion alone; one of these was approached with vitrectomy, the other with vitrectomy and lensectomy. Three traumatic perforating cases produced vitreous hemorrhage.

There was one case of massive unabsorbed vitreous hemorrhage secondary to hypertension.

Diabetic unabsorbed vitreous hemorrhage, requiring only vitrectomy, included ten patients.

There were twenty-four additional diabetic cases of vitreous hemorrhage and cataract requiring lensectomy and vitrectomy.

Fig. 8-22 shows a persistent fibrovascular stalk remnant after vitrectomy in a 30-year-old diabetic man (visual acuity 20/25). This patient had undergone an unsuccessful vitrectomy in his right eye a year earlier and a subsequent

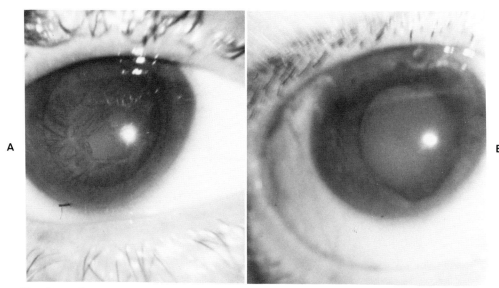

Fig. 8-20. Phacoemulsification postcataract membrane. **A,** Red reflex; **B,** postoperative appearance after use of the Roto-Extractor (red reflex).

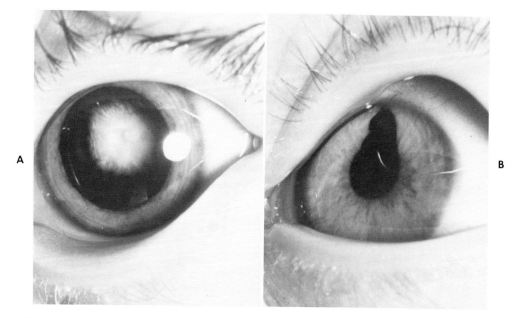

Fig. 8-21. A, Persistent hyperplastic primary vitreous 8 months old; **B,** postoperative appearance with inadvertent sector iridectomy.

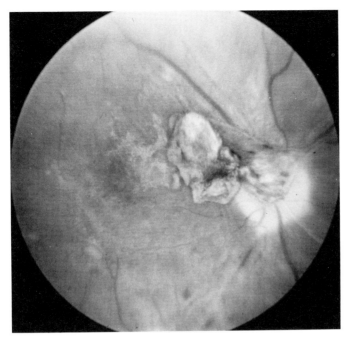

Fig. 8-22. Postoperative pars plana vitrectomy (20/25 visual acuity) with a residual fibrous retinitis proliferans stalk.

enucleation because of hemorrhage and glaucoma. His left eye had organized vitreous hemorrhage with good light projection in all quadrants. We performed a vitrectomy and cut and removed several layers of dense fibrous membranes. With a smooth blunt probe tip we then deflected the fibrous tissue to visualize the underlying retinal attachments. Two fibrous retinal attachments were noted, and we cut the fibrous band between the two to isolate them. An attachment to the disc was then severed, leaving a "morning glory" stalk emanating from the disc. Postoperative result one year later was 20/25.

Small vessels within fibrous retinitis proliferans can be severed and will not bleed significantly. If bleeding occurs, it can be controlled by raising the infusion pressure above the small capillary pressure so as to tamponade the bleeder. That is the importance of the closed vitrectomy system, namely, the ability to work in a pressurized eye. The goal in this type of surgery, in which membranes are cut or peeled, is to eliminate areas of twopoint traction that can give rise to subsequent shrinkage and detachment.

Fig. 8-23, A, shows a 93-year-old totally luxated lens after an attempted intracapsular cataract extraction with vitreous loss elsewhere. The patient had developed phacolytic glaucoma with a decompensated cornea. A pars plana incision was made, and cloudy opacified vitreous and lens cortex removed by the Roto-Extractor. An infusion Goldmann contact lens was then applied to the cornea to permit deeper visualization, and additional cortical material was re-

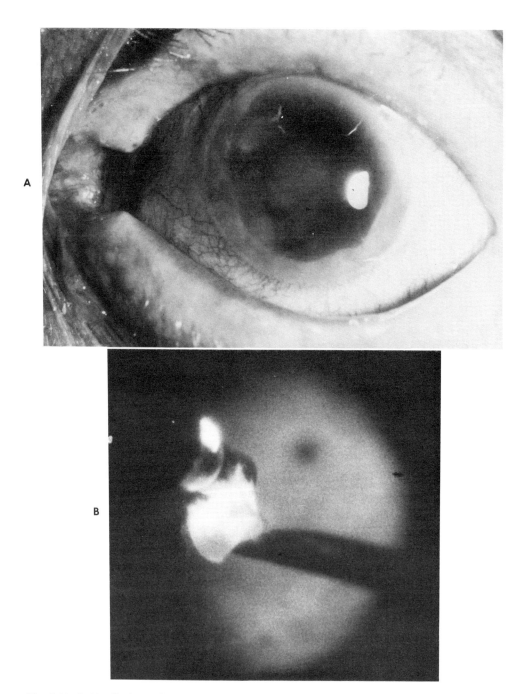

Fig. 8-23. A, Totally luxated cataract in a 93-year-old eye with phacolytic glaucoma and early corneal decompensation. The lens was dislocated posteriorly. **B,** Crushing the luxated lens fragment within the midvitreous cavity between the Roto-Extractor probe tip and a 21-gauge needle while packing the lens into the aspiration-cutting port.

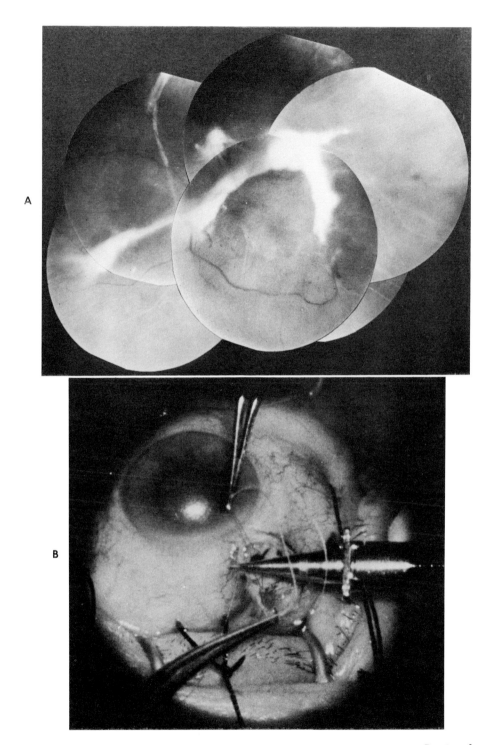

Continued.

Fig. 8-24. **A,** Collage of a preoperative diabetic retinitis proliferans with traction retinal detachment and a preretinal macular membrane or veil. **B,** Roto-Extractor trocar and cannula prepared for entry into the sclerotomy wound, everted by 7-0 Vicryl safety suture loops.

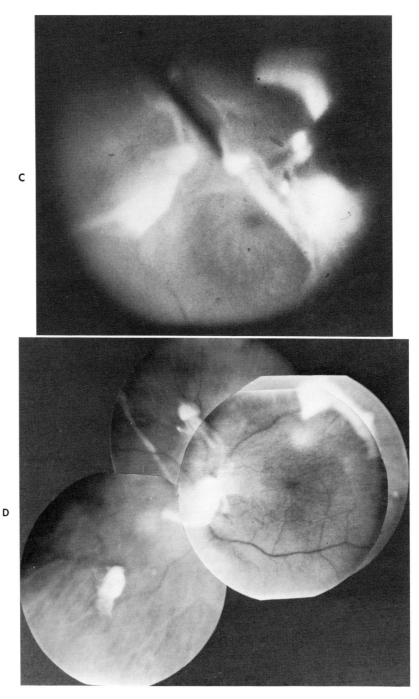

Fig. 8-24, cont'd. **C,** Two-instrument technique—a 22-gauge hooked needle peeling the premacular membrane or veil with Roto-Extractor fiber-optic illumination. **D,** Collage of a postoperative vitrectomy and membranectomy appearance (same patient).

moved down to the rock hard nucleus (too hard to aspirate). A 21-gauge needle was introduced through the opposite pars plana to crush the nucleus into the side cutter. Because of the long duty cycle and high-speed cutting with minimal interruption of vacuum, we were able to retain nuclear fragments in the mid-vitreous cavity without dropping them during cutter activation. The crushed fragments were picked up from the retinal surface, carried to the midvitreous cavity, and packed into the aspiration opening for engagement by the cutter blade (Fig. 8-23, *B*). All rigid lens fragments were thereby removed from the retinal surface.

I have had occasion to utilize this crushing technique five times thus far. All patients have done well, without complication; however, one cutter was ruined when the needle tip became stuck in the cutter opening.

Fig. 8-24, *A*, shows a traction detachment due to a diabetic fibrous retinitis proliferans with preretinal membrane veiling the macula. Two sclerotomy sites were prepared, one nasally and one temporally. The uvea within the sclerotomy was cauterized with a wet-field cautery to produce retraction, and a Vanas scissors was used to ensure that the opening through the uvea was adequate. A dilating trocar (Fig. 8-24, *B*) prepared a pathway for the Roto-Extractor probe tip with the fiber-optic light pipe. In this technique the opacified vitreous was first removed anteriorly. A 22-gauge straight needle on a syringe was then inserted through the superior nasal pars plana to prepare a pathway for the hooked 22-gauge needle used for membrane peeling. The preretinal membrane was then hooked and peeled from the macula (Fig. 8-24, *C*), and the fibrous ringlike arcade was fragmented and the material aspirated. This patient, 10 days after surgery, was able to read small newsprint with effort. The retina had flattened out (Fig. 8-24, *D*).

Table 8-2. Visual results in 100 consecutive Roto-Extractor operations

	Improved	*Not improved*	*Worse*
Congenital and developmental cataracts	12	0	0
Traumatic cataract	14	3	0
Cataracta complicata—uveitis	3	0	0
Hyphema with glaucoma	2	0	0
Complications of intracapsular cataract	15	3	1
Complications of Phacoemulsification	1	1	0
Persistent hyperplastic primary vitreous	1	0	0
Traumatic massive vitreous hemorrhage	1	2	2
Opaque vitreous and retinal detachment	2(1)°	0	0(1)°
Vitreous hemorrhage and branch vein occlusion	2(1)°	0(1)°	0
Hypertensive vitreous hemorrhage V (PP)	1	0	0
Diabetic vitreous hemorrhage V (PP)	6	2	2
Diabetic vitreous hemorrhage and cataract L & V (PP)	19	2	3

Code: ( )°, Late failure
PP, Pars plana approach
L, Lensectomy
V, Vitrectomy

The visual results of these 100 cases are shown in Table 8-2. The success rate in diabetics is fairly high. I should emphasize that I am very conservative and careful in case selection. Perhaps I have been too conservative, which would account for the high success rate.

EDITOR'S COMMENT

The individual case examples and illustrations used in this chapter were edited from an excellent 30-minute movie shown at the conference. The editor selected those cases which seemed to best illustrate the author's techniques and results.

9

Vitrectomy in diabetes and other disorders

RONALD G. MICHELS
STEPHEN J. RYAN, Jr.

Development of the pars plana vitrectomy technique using instruments with infusion, suction, and cutting features has opened new therapeutic avenues to a number of ocular disorders. Machemer,[13,15] Douvas,[2] and others[3,6-8,23,25,26] have introduced effective vitrectomy instruments; and Machemer[9-12,14,16] developed the surgical technique. With this technique opaque vitreous can be removed, intravitreal sheets and bands can be divided, and membranes can be peeled from the surface of the retina. Also the lens can be extracted, pupillary membranes excised, and vitreous removed from the anterior segment.

The ability to remove opaque vitreous and relieve vitreous traction is useful in the treatment of certain blinding complications of proliferative diabetic retinopathy, including vitreous hemorrhage and traction retinal detachment; however, this technique can be applied to a number of other ocular conditions as well:

1. Nonresolving vitreous opacities
2. Certain retinal detachments
    a. Traction detachments
    b. Certain giant tears
    c. Rhegmatogenous detachment and vitreous hemorrhage
    d. Rhegmatogenous detachment and vitreous traction
    e. Massive vitreous retraction (MVR)
3. Trauma
    a. Penetrating injuries of the posterior segment
    b. Nonmagnetic intraocular foreign bodies
4. Vitreous biopsy
5. Anterior segment reconstruction
6. Vitreous complications in the anterior segment
    a. Vitreous touch with corneal edema
    b. Aphakic pupillary block glaucoma
    c. Vitreous incarceration with persistent cystoid macular edema

7. Hemolytic, phacolytic, phacoanaphylactic glaucoma
8. Endophthalmitis
9. Other

NONRESOLVING VITREOUS OPACITIES

Blindness due to nonresolving vitreous opacities is the most common indication for pars plana vitreous surgery. The opacity is usually blood, although eyes with dense amyloid deposits or inflammatory debris in the vitreous are occasionally seen.

Proliferative diabetic retinopathy is the most common disorder leading to dense vitreous hemorrhage. Of our first 250 eyes undergoing pars plana vitrectomy, 50% were operated on for complications of diabetic retinopathy. Other disorders causing vitreous hemorrhage included old retinal branch-vein obstruction, Eales' disease, sickle hemoglobinopathies, and retinal tears with hemorrhage.

Early experience with vitrectomy demonstrated that the eye tolerates excision of formed vitreous surprisingly well. Opaque vitreous is easily identified; and with the aid of fiber-optic intraocular illumination,[24] all the formed vitreous can usually be excised except the anterior peripheral portion adjacent to the vitreous base. Exogenous solutions are used to replace the vitreous volume, and this fluid is rapidly replaced by aqueous humor. Creation of an optically clear vitreous cavity, filled with aqueous humor, permits improved vision in many eyes previously blinded by vitreous opacities.

The visual acuity following technically successful vitrectomy is limited by the functional capability of the retina. Usually the retina has been affected by the underlying disease, and postoperative vision is to some degree limited (Fig. 9-1). We have no way to reliably predict the potential level of retinal function in the presence of dense vitreous opacities. The level of visual acuity prior to vitreous hemorrhage is important, however, and the presence and quality of light projection are often our most reliable preoperative clinical tests. Preoperative evaluation by combined A- and B-scan ultrasonography[5] and bright-flash electroretinography (ERG)[12] is of value in determining the presence and degree of retinal detachment; but the final decision regarding a recommendation for vitrectomy is based largely on clinical findings, the potential for significant benefit to the individual patient, and the attendant risks of surgery.

Results of vitrectomy performed for nonresolving opacities vary with the underlying disease process. We have reviewed 125 consecutive vitrectomies performed at the Wilmer Institute between November, 1973, and January, 1975. Average follow-up was 8 months, with a minimum follow-up of 3 months. In nondiabetic patients ten of twelve eyes (83%) achieved improved vision. In diabetic patients with vitreous hemorrhage but without significant traction detachment, vision improved in sixteen of twenty-three eyes (70%). In diabetic patients with both dense vitreous hemorrhage and traction detachment involving the posterior retina, vision increased in nineteen of thirty-six eyes (53%).

The postoperative visual acuity in eyes with improved vision varied from

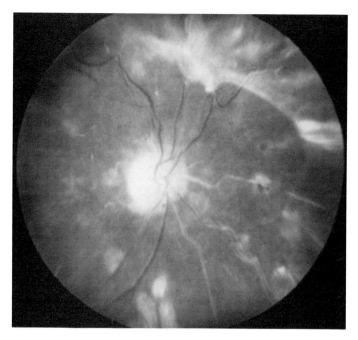

Fig. 9-1. Pale optic nerve and sheathed retinal vessels after vitrectomy to remove long-standing vitreous hemorrhage in a patient with proliferative diabetic retinopathy. Vision improved to only 3/200 because of occlusive retinal vascular disease.

20/20 to 3/200. Few diabetic patients achieved final vision of 20/50 or better—especially if significant traction retinal detachment was present preoperatively. Five of sixteen diabetic eyes with improved vision and without significant traction detachment obtained final vision of 20/50 or better. Fourteen of these sixteen eyes achieved final vision of 20/300 or better. When both vitreous hemorrhage and significant traction detachment were present preoperatively, only two of nineteen diabetic eyes with improved vision postoperatively achieved vision of 20/50 or better. Eleven of the nineteen eyes attained final vision of 20/300 or better.

Despite a low level of final measurable acuity, many patients were substantially helped by moderate improvement in vision permitting a greater degree of unaided mobility and independence.

CERTAIN RETINAL DETACHMENTS

Pars plana vitreous surgery is useful in the treatment of certain complicated retinal detachments. It is of special value in treating nonrhegmatogenous traction detachments and retinal tears greater than 180° with a folded-over retinal flap. It can be combined with scleral buckling to treat detachments complicated by dense vitreous hemorrhage, detachments with severe vitreous traction, and detachments complicated by early massive vitreous retraction (MVR).

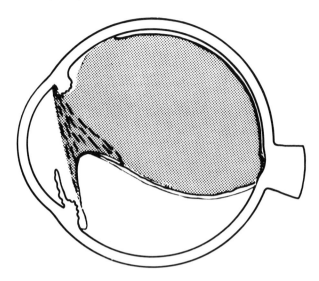

Fig. 9-2. Vitreous sheet incarcerated in a cataract wound, causing extensive detachment of the inferior retina and ciliary epithelium. (From Norton, E. W. D., and Machemer, R.: Am. J. Ophthalmol. **72:**705, 1971.)

Traction detachments

Vitreous traction may cause retinal detachment without retinal breaks; and the detachment can usually be cured by cutting the vitreous bands, thereby releasing the traction. Nonrhegmatogenous traction retinal detachment may occur as a complication of vitreous incarcerated in a cataract wound, or it may follow a penetrating injury of the posterior segment.

Though the most common cause of traction detachment is proliferative diabetic retinopathy, other proliferative retinopathies may also cause such detachments.

Vitreous sheets incarcerated in a cataract wound can contract postoperatively and cause traction on the inferior vitreous base with detachment of the inferior retina and adjacent ciliary epithelium (Fig. 9-2.) This condition is difficult to treat by conventional scleral buckling techniques because the traction tends to be progressive. Surgery is indicated when the detachment is extensive and threatens the posterior retina. Norton and Machemer[22] first described the successful use of vitreous surgery to cut these sheets and release the traction. They noted, furthermore, that scleral buckling may be necessary because of secondary changes in the inferior vitreous base and retina. We have also combined pars plana vitrectomy with scleral buckling in eyes with vitreous incarcerated in a cataract wound to successfully treat progressive detachment that threatened the macula.

Traction detachments of varying complexity may complicate penetrating injuries of the posterior segment. Transvitreal sheets and bands often develop along the path of the penetrating injury, causing traction on the adjacent retina

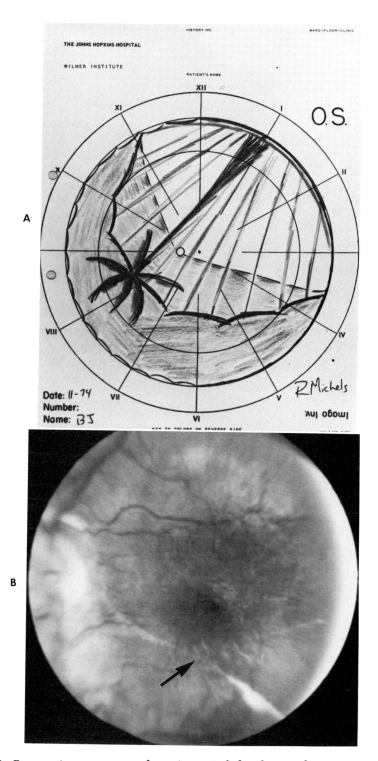

Fig. 9-3. A, Preoperative appearance of traction retinal detachment after penetrating injury with a dart. The posterior penetration site is in the inferonasal quadrant. A broad vitreous sheet causes extensive retinal detachment, impinging on the macula. B, Postoperative appearance after successful retinal reattachment by cutting the vitreous sheet and scleral buckling. The old demarcation line is present just inferior to the macula (arrow).

or on the vitreous base 180° away and resulting in traction detachment; or subsequent retinal tears (including giant breaks) may cause rhegmatogenous detachment. Unfortunately the retina frequently becomes involved in a fibrous scar, which makes successful reattachment difficult. A combination of vitreous surgery to cut the traction bands and scleral buckling to support segments of permanently distorted and contracted retina permits successful reattachment in selected cases (Fig. 9-3).

Traction retinal detachment often complicates proliferative diabetic retinopathy. The posterior vitreous is attached to sites of epiretinal proliferation and may result in traction detachment of the underlying retina. Characteristically detachment occurs along the course of the temporal vascular arcades, but other areas may be involved. Vitreous surgery should be considered if the macula has been recently detached, with a significant decrease in vision (Fig. 9-4). Extensive detachment along the vascular arcades often spares the macula; because of the operative risks in these eyes, we do not recommend vitreous surgery before the macula is detached.

Diabetic eyes with traction detachment demonstrate vitreoretinal relationships of widely varying complexity. In some eyes the posterior hyaloid is only minimally separated from the retina—with large areas of vitreoretinal adhesion, extensive retinal detachment, and prominent growth of new blood vessels along the posterior hyaloid. This situation is most often seen in juvenile diabetics dur-

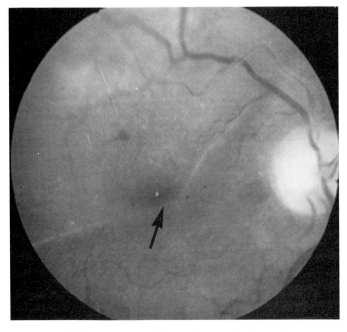

Fig. 9-4. Traction retinal detachment involving the macula (arrow) in a patient with proliferative diabetic retinopathy and recent decrease in vision.

ing an active phase of neovascular proliferation with rapidly progressive traction detachments. These eyes present severe technical problems during surgery because of the difficulty in separating the vitreoretinal adhesions and the tendency of fragile new blood vessels to bleed. Two-instrument techniques, as described by Machemer,[11] are required; and, despite extreme care, inadvertent retinal breaks may be created. A tendency for postoperative bleeding and a high risk of rubeosis iridis make these eyes poor surgical candidates.

Other diabetic eyes show extensive collapse of the vitreous, with a funnel-shaped configuration of the posterior hyaloid extending from the vitreous base to areas of vitreoretinal adhesion posteriorly (Fig. 9-5). Cutting this circumferential vitreous sheet releases traction on the posterior retina and allows traction retinal detachment to flatten. All vitreous attachments between the posterior retina and the vitreous base must be cut, and vitreous bands bridging sites of vitreoretinal adhesion must be divided. If these sheets are not cut, they tend to contract postoperatively and result in increased traction. A transparent membrane of taut cortical vitreous often bridges the macula, extending between the superior and inferior vascular arcades. It can be divided using a hooked needle as described by Machemer.[11] Although the presence of epiretinal membranes may prevent full

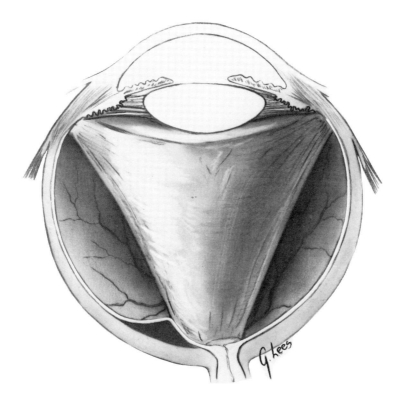

Fig. 9-5. Funnel-shaped configuration of the posterior hyaloid after collapse of the vitreous Traction extends from the vitreous base anteriorly to the optic nerve and posteriorly to areas of vitreoretinal adhesion, causing retinal detachment.

reattachment in some areas—when vitreous traction has been released, the retina tends to reattach rapidly.

These complex vitreoretinal relationships and areas of traction retinal detachment are most often encountered after removal of vitreous opacities in diabetic eyes blinded by massive hemorrhage. Although vision seldom improves to better than 20/200 if the macula has been detached for a prolonged time, anatomic reattachment of the retina is usually possible. We have operated on three other eyes with clear media and progressive traction detachment involving the posterior retina. In each case the macula had been detached for several months; and despite successful reattachment of the retina, vision did not improve postoperatively.

Certain giant retinal tears

Giant retinal tears with folded-over flaps that cannot be unfolded by preoperative or intraoperative positioning are generally not successfully repaired using conventional techniques. Vitreous traction on the edge of the tear, or formed vitreous between the retina and the pigment epithelium, may prevent the flap from unfolding (Fig. 9-6). Vitrectomy is used to relieve vitreous traction and

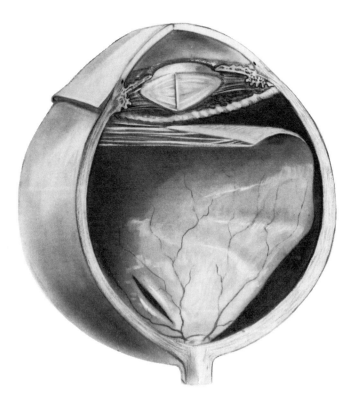

Fig. 9-6. Complicated retinal detachment with vitreous traction on the edge of a 150° tear and a linear posterior retinal break extending within two disc diameters of the optic nerve. Retinal reattachment was achieved by vitrectomy, scleral buckling, and intraocular gas injection.

remove formed vitreous, permitting the flap to be mobilized and positioned against the pigment epithelium. Also removal of formed vitreous creates a fluid space in which a gas bubble can be placed for internal tamponade and from which fluid can be released to permit raising a scleral buckle.

Machemer and Norton[14] developed a technique to unfold retinal flaps using a combination of vitrectomy, intraoperative positioning with a rotating table, and gas injection to mechanically unfold the retina. With this technique the entire vitreous cavity is filled with gas; and as the retina unfolds, it is reattached and held against the pigment epithelium by the intravitreal bubble. The authors find the technique especially useful in treating tears of more than 180°; tears less than 180° can usually be treated with vitrectomy and a smaller intraocular gas bubble, using postoperative postioning to unfold the retina. With this technique it is not necessary to turn the patient upside down during the operative procedure.[21] We have used a combination of vitrectomy, scleral buckling, and intraocular gas to successfully treat one eye with 150° giant tear complicated by vitreous traction on the edge of the tear.

Rhegmatogenous detachment and vitreous hemorrhage

Certain rhegmatogenous detachments complicated by dense vitreous hemorrhage can be successfully treated using a combination of pars plana vitrectomy and scleral buckling. Vitreous hemorrhage associated with acute retinal tears is usually mild but may initially obscure visualization of the retina. Bilateral patching and bed rest with the head elevated often result in settling of the blood, permitting identification and treatment of retinal breaks. Massive vitreous hemorrhage, however, is occasionally associated with retinal tears and detachment. The diagnosis of detachment can be confirmed by ultrasonography and bright-flash ERG. If the blood does not clear, a retinal reattachment operation without intraocular visualization can be performed—including extensive diathermy or cryotherapy, a broad circumferential scleral buckle, and drainage of subretinal fluid.

We have used pars plana vitrectomy to clear the vitreous blood, thus permitting identification of retinal breaks and allowing appropriate scleral buckling during the same operation. Also a gas bubble is placed in the vitreous cavity to tamponade the retinal breaks and assure postoperative settling of the retina.[19,20] Vitreous surgery is especially hazardous in the presence of both vitreous blood and retinal detachment, and extreme caution is required to prevent cutting the retina. The infusion pressure is maintained at a low level, and intermittent back-pressure through the suction line is used if the retina approaches the cutting port.

Rhegmatogenous detachment and vitreous traction

Rhegmatogenous retinal detachment may be complicated by severe vitreous traction which prevents settling of the retina and closure of retinal breaks when treated by conventional scleral buckling techniques. Vitrectomy will relieve the traction and allow the retina to settle. Also, after vitrectomy, intraocular gas can be conveniently used to create an internal tamponade and assure settling of the retina. When intraocular gas is used, the subretinal fluid does not have to be drained—thereby eliminating one potentially hazardous step in the operation.[19] Vitrectomy adds a special risk to the procedure, however, and is reserved for reoperation on eyes in which vitreous traction caused failure of a conventional buckling procedure. We have successfully used a combination of vitrectomy, cryotherapy, scleral buckling, and the intraocular injection of gas in three such cases.

Massive vitreous retraction

The role of pars plana vitrectomy in retinal detachment complicated by massive vitreous retraction (MVR) is uncertain. In these eyes the retina is highly elevated and held in rigid folds by transvitreal traction and contracture of a cellular epiretinal membrane. Retinal breaks thus cannot flatten on a scleral buckle; and when the process is advanced, this condition is virtually inoperable by conventional techniques.

Successful reattachment in cases of MVR is dependent on mobilizing the folds of retina. This can be accomplished by cutting the transvitreal traction sheets and peeling the epiretinal membrane off the retina with the two-instrument technique of Machemer.[11,12] If the process is of relatively recent onset, cutting and peeling can be done relatively easily. In eyes with long-standing detachment and MVR, however, the membrane is firmly adherent to the inner retina and cannot be mechanically separated. Therefore vitreous surgery may have a role only in certain eyes with recent-onset MVR. We have successfully reattached the retina in a 15-month-old patient with MVR complicating a giant tear. A high scleral buckle, generous cryotherapy, and intraocular gas were used after vitreous surgery was first performed to mobilize the fixed retina.

TRAUMA

The pars plana vitrectomy technique offers a new approach to management of certain penetrating injuries of the posterior segment and selected intraocular foreign bodies.

Penetrating injuries of the posterior segment

Penetrating injuries cause varying amounts of initial mechanical damage and may be complicated later by fibrous ingrowth, vitreous traction-band formation, and complex retinal detachment. In eyes with recent penetrating injury that largely spares the cornea, the vitrectomy technique is useful to remove a cataractous lens, excise vitreous from the anterior segment, and remove vitreous blood thereby permitting treatment of retinal breaks or detachment before intraocular organization leads to inoperable damage.

Early vitrectomy prevents certain complications of late vitreous organization. Vitrectomy is a potentially dangerous procedure, however, and should be used only when conservative management is likely to fail. We employ early vitrectomy in eyes with an admixture of lens material and vitreous in which severe inflammation and organization are certain to follow. Also in eyes with dense vitreous hemorrhage and evidence of retinal damage, early vitrectomy is used to clear the opacities—permitting treatment of retinal breaks or detachment. In eyes with clear media, vitrectomy is used only if vitreous traction bands develop and result in retinal detachment. Frequent observation is required in these eyes because the retina may become involved in a fibrous scar, causing permanent distortion and making successful reattachment difficult. Finally, we occasionally use the vitrectomy technique in severely traumatized eyes with light perception vision when enucleation is being considered to prevent possible sympathetic ophthalmia.

We "explore" the eye by vitrectomy and if the posterior segment is found to be damaged beyond hope of salvage proceed with enucleation during the same operation.

Early vitrectomy after penetrating trauma prevents the later development of transvitreal traction bands. These patients are often young, however, and the posterior hyaloid may not be separated from the retina. Therefore it may be difficult to remove all the cortical vitreous; and although transvitreal sheets are absent, this remaining vitreous may later contract and cause puckering of the retina.

Finally, it must be noted that less than six years of follow-up are available on the earliest cases of pars plana vitrectomy. How long these eyes will continue to function well after vitreous excision is not known. Because many such traumatized eyes are in young patients, we believe vitrectomy should be reserved for eyes that otherwise are likely to be lost. We do not use vitrectomy as a prophylactic measure to prevent possible traction-band formation.

Selected intraocular foreign bodies

The pars plana vitrectomy technique, combined with the use of specialized intraocular forceps, has dramatically changed the management of certain intraocular foreign bodies. Machemer[11] developed this new technique, which permits forceps extraction of nonmagnetic foreign bodies from the posterior segment under visual control after any lens or vitreous opacities have been removed. Nonmagnetic foreign bodies may pose a threat to the eye in several respects—mechanical damage by the penetrating injury, toxicity from the foreign-body material, infection, and secondary changes in the vitreous that may lead to retinal detachment or other complications. Previously no method was available to clear vitreous opacities to permit direct visualization and extraction of the foreign body or to prevent secondary vitreous complications related to the entry or removal of the foreign body.

The surgical technique includes an initial peritomy and exposure as used in retinal reattachment surgery. A double Flieringa ring is sutured to the globe (Fig. 9-7, A). This ring maintains normal configuration of the anterior segment, permitting use of a corneal contact lens during extraction of the foreign body

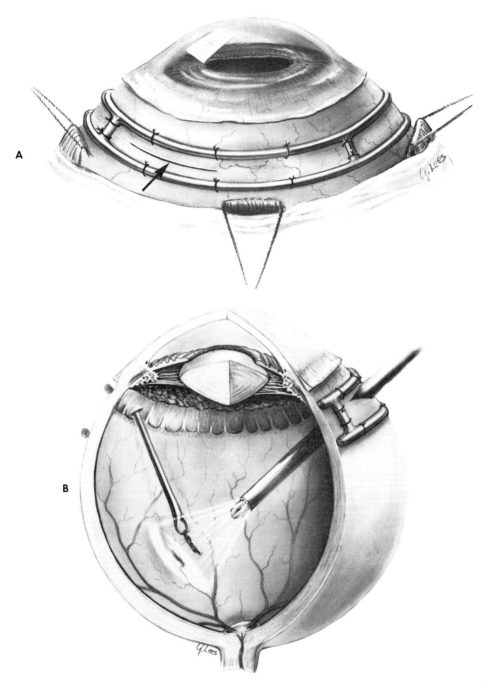

Fig. 9-7. A, Double Flieringa ring used to support the globe during extraction of an intra-vitreal foreign body. A long pars plana incision (arrow) may be required to permit with-drawal of the foreign body (held by forceps). **B,** Two-instrument technique for extraction of a nonmagnetic intravitreal foreign body. The vitrectomy instrument is used to clear vitreous opacities, mobilize the foreign body, and illuminate the operative field. The foreign body is grasped with special forceps. (From Michels, R. G.: Arch. Ophthalmol. **93**:1003, 1975.)

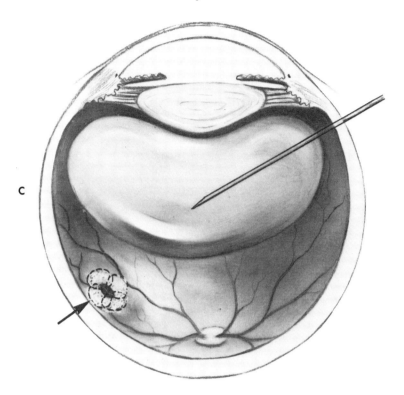

Fig. 9-7, cont'd. C, After vitrectomy and removal of the intravitreal foreign body, any retinal break can be treated with cryotherapy (arrow) and a gas bubble injected to tamponade the retinal break. (From Michels, R. G.: Arch. Ophthalmol. **93:**1003, 1975.)

when there may be extreme hypotony.[17] The vitrectomy instrument is used to remove the lens if it is cataractous and to clear any vitreous opacities. As much formed vitreous as possible is removed to prevent later traction-band formation. The foreign body is mobilized with the vitrectomy instrument and extracted with forceps through a separate pars plana incision (Fig. 9-7, *B*). The fiberoptic sleeve of the vitrectomy instrument provides optimum reflex-free illumination. Any retinal breaks may be treated by cryotherapy, with or without scleral buckling. A gas bubble is placed in the vitreous cavity, and postoperative positioning is used to tamponade the retinal breaks against the treated pigment epithelium (Fig. 9-7, *C*).

We have employed this technique in four eyes with nonmagnetic intraocular foreign bodies in the vitreous and in one eye with a magnetic foreign body whose size and configuration were such that forceps extraction seemed advisable. Our first case was a 13-year-old boy who was injured by an exploding soft-drink bottle and had a large (13×3×3 mm) glass foreign body in the vitreous (Fig. 9-8, *A*). The glass was removed using this technique, and 9 months later the vision was 20/30 and the eye stable (Fig. 9-8, *B*). In four of our five cases, the foreign body was successfully removed and the eye salvaged with good vision

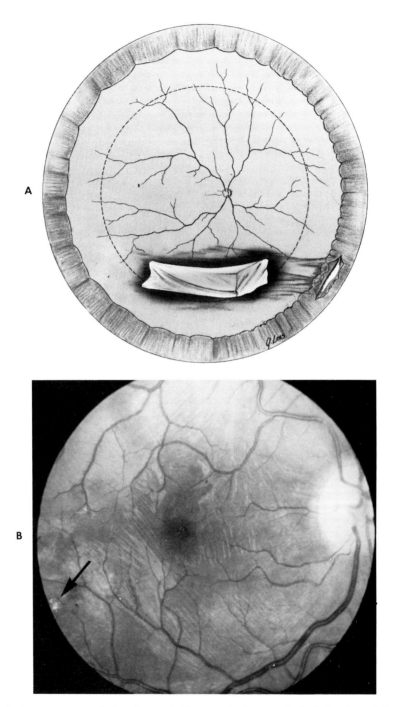

Fig. 9-8. A, Large intravitreal glass foreign body caused when a soft-drink bottle exploded. The foreign body was removed by the two-instrument technique of Machemer. **B,** Fundus appearance 6 months after removal of the glass foreign body. The scar temporal to the macula (arrow) is the site of the sealed retinal break.

Table 9-1. Intraocular foreign bodies

Case no.	Preoperative vision	Postoperative vision	Comments	Follow-up (mo.)
1	8/200	20/30	Large glass foreign body in vitreous	12
2	HM 2 ft	20/15	Three lead foreign bodies vitritis, cataract	12
3	HM 1 ft	20/50	No. 6 lead shot, vitritis, cataract	12
4	20/400	20/40	Nail impaled in retina and sclera	9
5	HM 2 ft	5/200	Lead foreign body under retina, not removed	6

(Table 9-1). In the fifth case the foreign body proved to be lodged under the retina and could not be extracted despite an ab externo approach. Although the foreign body remained intraocular, the retina was successfully reattached. In one eye the lens was not damaged by the initial injury and was left in place during the foreign-body extraction.

VITREOUS BIOPSY

Vitreous biopsy may be indicated to establish a diagnosis in eyes with a progressive infectious, inflammatory, or infiltrative process involving the vitreous. The most frequent indications for vitreous biopsy are possible mycotic endophthalmitis and ocular reticulum cell sarcoma. Mycotic endophthalmitis may present with white "fluff" balls in the vitreous several weeks after cataract surgery or as the first sign of widespread systemic fungal involvement in debilitated or immuneincompetent patients. Differential diagnosis on clinical grounds may be difficult, especially when dealing with a late postoperative infection in an eye that has been treated with antibiotics prophylactically. Bacterial endophthalmitis partially suppressed by antibiotic therapy may form localized abscesses within the vitreous, giving a clinical appearance similar to that of fungus lesions. Maximum accuracy of diagnosis is important to permit choice of appropriate antibiotic or antimycotic therapy, especially before beginning a long and potentially toxic course of antimycotic medication.

Reticulum cell sarcoma may present with ocular involvement that has features similar to those of uveitis—including aqueous flare and cells, vitreous cells, and retinal or subretinal infiltrate. This condition usually occurs in patients over age 40, and there may be evidence of systemic disease (although in some patients the eye is the only apparent site of involvement). Characteristically there is infiltration of the choroid and retina with tumor cells, and the tumor cells may also migrate into the vitreous.[1] Clinically the vitreous shows accumulation of gray debris lining the vitreous fibrils (Fig. 9-9). Vitreous involvement may be so dense that visualization of the fundus is impaired and vision significantly re-

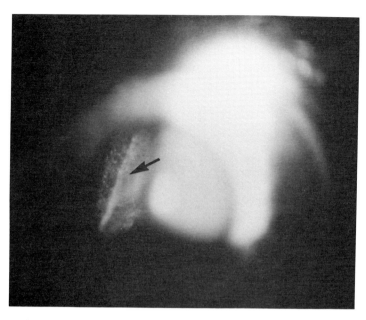

Fig. 9-9. Slit lamp appearance of an ocular reticulum cell sarcoma involving the vitreous. Dense gray opacities line the vitreous fibrils (arrow). (From Michels, R. G.: Arch. Ophthalmol. **93**:1331, 1975.)

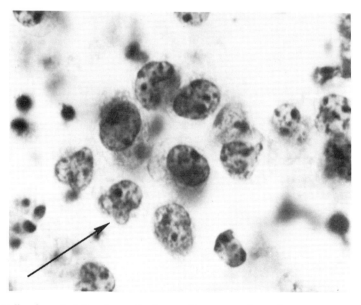

Fig. 9-10. Cells characteristic of a reticulum cell sarcoma from the vitreous of the patient illustrated in Fig. 9-9. Cytologic features include thin scanty cytoplasm, nuclei with prominent nucleoli, and nuclei with distinctive fingerlike protrusions (arrow) (modified Papanicolaou stain ×1500). (From Michels, R. G.: Arch. Ophthalmol. **93**:1331, 1975.)

duced. Inflammatory cells may be present in the anterior segment, but tumor cells have not been demonstrated in the aqueous.

The pars plana vitrectomy technique permits controlled biopsy of intravitreal lesions under direct visualization and microscopic control. The excised material remains sterile and can be removed from the suction syringe for culture and cytologic examination. Cellular morphology is well preserved, and cellular content of the specimen can be concentrated by passing the material through a Millipore filter.

We have successfully used this technique to identify the organism in one case of suspected mycotic endophthalmitis and to establish the diagnosis of reticulum cell sarcoma in two patients presenting with ocular involvement (Fig. 9-10).[18] In both the latter cases vision improved from removal of the considerable vitreous opacities. We have not encountered complications in these few cases of vitrectomy done for diagnostic purposes.

ANTERIOR SEGMENT RECONSTRUCTION

Vitrectomy instrumentation and techniques can be applied to several difficult surgical problems of the anterior segment. We have found this approach particularly useful in selected eyes with an occluded or inadequate pupillary space due to dense membranous cataracts, vascularized pupillary membranes, secluded and/or updrawn pupils, and persistent hyperplastic primary vitreous (PHPV). The vitrectomy instrument can create a pupillary space by excising dense fibrous material that is too tough to be cut with a knife.

Although a limbus entry site may be used in selected cases, we generally introduce the vitrectomy instrument through the pars plana. Light from the fiber-optic sleeve shows the position of the instrument tip through an opaque pupillary membrane. Iris tissue and soft pliable membranes are readily excised, a bit at a time, until an adequate pupillary space is created. Tough nonpliable membranes often cannot be aspirated into the cutting port, and a two-instrument technique is used to cut the membrane into wedge-shaped sections. A knife is introduced into the anterior chamber through peripheral clear cornea and is used to cut the membrane against the instrument tip posteriorly. The sections of membrane are aspirated into the cutting port and excised (Fig. 9-11).

We have operated on nine eyes with dense fibrotic capsulolenticular membranes (membranous cataracts) using this technique. In each case an adequate pupillary space was created (Fig. 9-12). Vision improved postoperatively in every eye; seven of the nine eyes achieved final vision of 20/40 or better. Preexisting macular damage and congenital nystagmus resulted in final vision of less than 20/40 in two eyes. No intraoperative complications occurred, but two patients developed retinal detachment later due to round holes remote from the sclerotomy site. (Both detachments were successfully repaired.)

Opaque vascularized pupillary membranes may occur as a complication of anterior segment inflammation or total hyphema. The membrane can be excised with the vitrectomy instrument, and the cataractous lens removed in phakic

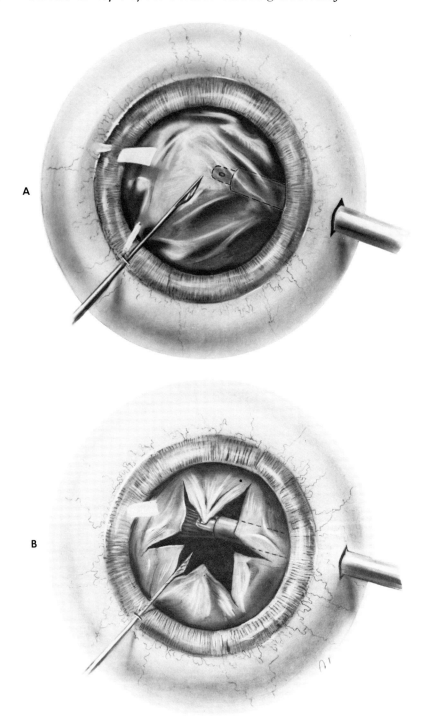

Fig. 9-11. A, Two-instrument technique for cutting a nonpliable pupillary membrane. The vitrectomy instrument tip supports the membrane from behind and serves as a chopping block while the membrane is cut with a knife. **B,** Portions of the pupillary membrane are excised with the vitrectomy instrument after having been cut by the two-instrument technique.

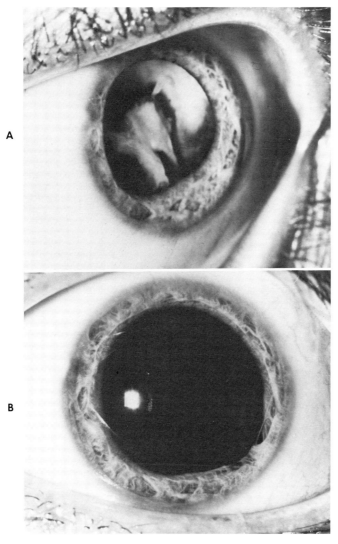

Fig. 9-12. **A,** Preoperative appearance of a membranous cataract seventeen years after penetrating injury with a paper clip. **B,** Postoperative appearance. There is a large clear pupillary
space 6 weeks after excision of the membranous cataract by the pars plana technique.

eyes (Fig. 9-13). Bleeding from iris neovascularization is stopped by elevating
the intraocular pressure. We have successfully operated on two such cases, and
vision improved postoperatively. A postoperative hyphema complicated one
case, but this cleared rapidly.

Secluded and/or updrawn pupils may require surgery to create an adequate
pupillary space for visual purposes or to relieve iris bombé with secondary
glaucoma. We have operated on two eyes with inadequate updrawn pupils and
on one eye with a secluded pupil and iris bombé. A large pupillary space was

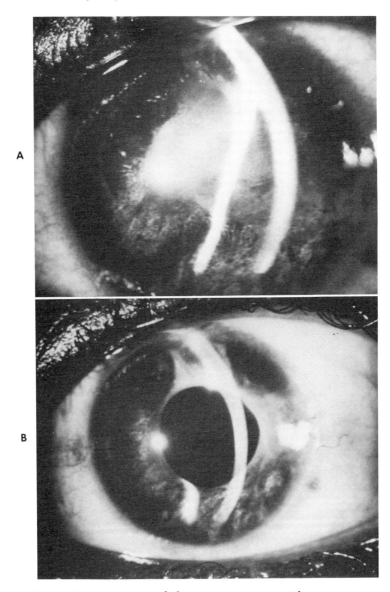

Fig. 9-13. A, Preoperative appearance of the anterior segment with a mature cataract, vascularized pupillary membrane, and shallow anterior chamber after blunt trauma and total hyphema. **B,** Postoperative appearance after excision of the pupillary membrane and removal of the cataract by the pars plana technique. The anterior chamber is of normal depth.

achieved in each case and the iris bombé was relieved (Fig. 9-14). No complications occurred and vision improved in each case.

We have successfully used the vitrectomy technique to aspirate the cataractous lens and excise the retrolenticular membrane in one eye with PHPV. This congenital anomaly is usually monocular and characterized by microphthalmos and a retrolenticular fibrovascular membrane with traction on the ciliary pro-

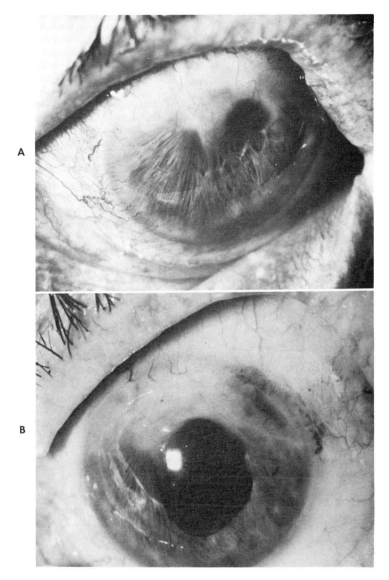

Fig. 9-14. A, Preoperative appearance of an eye with inadequate updrawn pupil after vitreous loss during cataract surgery. **B,** Postoperative appearance after a large pupillary space was created by the pars plana vitrectomy technique.

cesses. The condition often results in cataract formation and progressive flattening of the anterior chamber. Early lens aspiration and discission or excision of the retrolenticular membrane may prevent loss of the eye, but dense form vision amblyopia usually limits the visual function.

We have used the vitrectomy technique to successfully remove the cataract and excise the retrolenticular membrane in one eye with PHPV. A limbus entry site was chosen to avoid possible damage to the retina in the small eye. A technically successful result was achieved without complications. This was an unusual case with bilateral PHPV; and although the child is too young for acuity measurement, vision has seemed good with a contact lens. (The fellow eye was initially operated on by conventional techniques which resulted in an inadequate pupil with iris bombé that subsequently required additional surgery.)

VITREOUS COMPLICATIONS IN THE ANTERIOR SEGMENT

Pars plana vitrectomy techniques can be applied to certain vitreous complications in the anterior segment—vitreous touch with corneal edema, aphakic pupillary block glaucoma, and vitreous incarceration in a cataract wound with persistent cystoid macular edema.

Vitreous touch with corneal edema

In aphakic eyes formed vitreous may herniate into the anterior chamber and come into contact with the central corneal endothelium. This can damage the endothelium and result in persistent corneal edema and ocular irritation. Corneal damage is most likely to occur if central corneal guttatae are present. Formed vitreous is readily removed from the anterior chamber by the pars plana vitrectomy technique; and if permanent endothelial damage has not already occurred, the cornea clears.

The instrument tip is placed in the pupillary space with the cutting port directed anteriorly. Vitreous is gently aspirated from the anterior chamber and is replaced by infusion from the vitrectomy instrument without collapse of the cornea. The vitreous peels off the corneal endothelium, and all visible vitreous can be removed from the anterior chamber. Additional formed vitreous is excised behind the iris plane to prevent postoperative herniation into the anterior chamber. We have operated on two such patients—and there was postoperative clearing of the corneal edema with decreased ocular irritation.

Aphakic pupillary block glaucoma

In aphakic eyes formed vitreous occasionally obstructs the pupillary space and iridectomy sites—resulting in pooling of aqueous posteriorly, shallowing of the anterior chamber, and angle closure glaucoma (aphakic pupillary block glaucoma).

When the pupillary block cannot be relieved by medical therapy, surgery is required. Incision of the anterior hyaloid face often relieves the obstruction but may be complicated by vitreous to the corneal wound or reformation of the hyaloid face with recurrence of pupillary block. The vitrectomy technique can be used to permanently relieve the pupillary block and remove all vitreous from the anterior chamber.

The instrument tip is introduced through the pars plana and positioned in the pupillary space. Gentle suction brings the bulging hyaloid face to the cutting port, where it is incised. This relieves the pupillary block and results in immediate deepening of the anterior chamber.

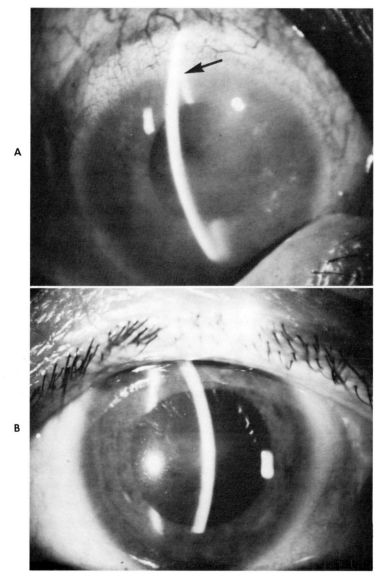

Fig. 9-15. A, Preoperative appearance of an eye with aphakic pupillary block glaucoma. The anterior chamber is shallow centrally and flat peripherally (arrow). **B,** Postoperative appearance after relief of the pupillary block and excision of formed vitreous by the pars plana vitrectomy technique. The anterior chamber is of normal depth centrally, and no vitreous is present in the anterior segment.

The remaining vitreous face is excised along with additional formed vitreous behind the iris plane. An attempt is made to separate the synechiae between the anterior vitreous face and the iris pigment epithelium by grasping the vitreous with suction and peeling it away from the iris. This results in a normal-appearing anterior chamber free of formed vitreous.

We have used the pars plana vitrectomy technique in four eyes with aphakic pupillary block glaucoma. In each case the anterior chamber deepened dramatically and no complications occurred (Fig. 9-15). In three of the four eyes, however, the anterior chamber had been flat for more than 10 days and extensive peripheral anterior synechiae persisted, resulting in secondary glaucoma. The technical results in these cases have been encouraging. Nevertheless, comparing the vitrectomy technique with the simpler discission method of treating this condition, we believe the pars plana approach introduces additional surgical risks and a longer follow-up with evaluation of complications is necessary.

Vitreous incarceration with persistent cystoid macular edema

Cystoid macular edema is a nonspecific maculopathy characterized by leakage from the perifoveal capillary bed of the retina causing cystlike accumulation of edema in the outer half of the retina. This maculopathy occurs in association with a number of retinal vascular disorders and ocular inflammatory conditions. It also follows various kinds of ophthalmic surgery. Its etiology is unknown; but the presence of cystoid edema in conditions associated with inflammation or surgical trauma suggests that intraocular irritation can disturb the permeability characteristics of the perifoveal capillaries, resulting in leakage of fluid.

Cystoid macular edema after cataract surgery (the Irvine-Gass syndrome) occurs commonly. The incidence, however, seems to be increased when vitreous is incarcerated in the wound. The macular edema usually clears spontaneously but may persist and cause significant visual loss. In our experience persistent cystoid macular edema is often associated with vitreous incarcerated in the limbus wound and chronic intraocular inflammation.

Attempts have been made to free the incarcerated vitreous, and Iliff[4] has reported improved vision when the vitreous bands were cut. Single bands can be divided with a knife or scissors, but broad vitreous sheets usually require reopening the limbus incision and anterior vitrectomy. We have used the pars plana vitrectomy technique to cut broad vitreous sheets in selected cases of cystoid macular edema persisting for more than one year. Fiber-optic intraocular illumination permits identification of the sheet, which is cut in the pupillary space. Portions of the sheet extending from the superior vitreous base and wrapping around the pupillary margin are elevated with a knife and displaced into the pupillary space to be cut (Fig. 9-16).

We have operated in five such cases and have successfully removed all vitreous from the wound in four of the five (Fig. 9-17). No complications have occurred. In one eye the macular edema subsided and vision improved from 20/100

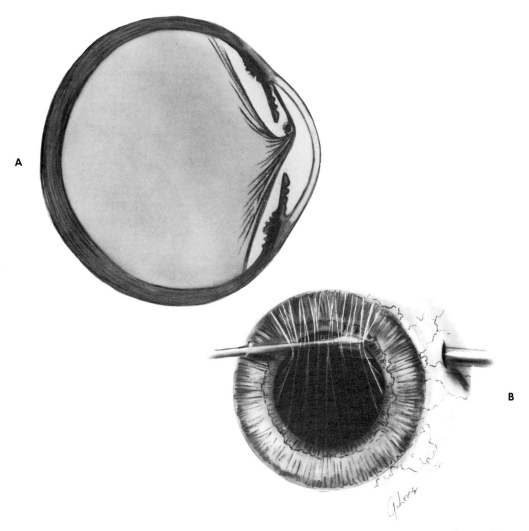

Fig. 9-16. A, Vitreous incarcerated in a cataract wound is elevated from the iris surface with a knife and displaced into the pupillary space. **B,** The vitreous sheet is cut with the vitrectomy instrument, releasing traction on both the superior and the inferior vitreous base.

to 20/25 during the subsequent 6 months. In two eyes edema and vision remained unchanged one year after vitrectomy. In the two remaining eyes follow-up has been too short to assess the results.

Although it is possible to excise vitreous from the wound, we are presently uncertain as to whether persistent cystoid macular edema is an indication for vitrectomy. Our early results are equivocal, and the etiology of the edema is not understood. Our intention has been to release traction on the vitreous base and adjacent ciliary body by cutting the taut vitreous sheets. This could result in less intraocular irritation and stabilize the permeability characteristics of the perifoveal capillary bed.

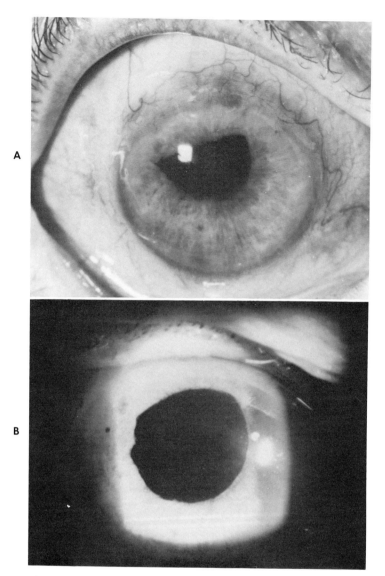

Fig. 9-17. A, Preoperative appearance of an updrawn pupil caused by a broad vitreous sheet incarcerated in the limbus wound superiorly. **B,** Postoperative appearance of the eye, with a rounded pupil, after the vitreous sheet was excised by the pars plana vitrectomy technique.

EDITOR'S NOTE

As the authors have stipulated, the benefits of pars plana vitrectomy in the I-G syndrome are presently not known. When one considers the fact that this condition is relatively common (both with and without vitreous incarceration), it becomes evident that a proper prospective controlled study should be undertaken to determine the efficacy of vitrectomy in eyes with cystoid macular edema of at least one year's duration.

HEMOLYTIC, PHACOLYTIC, AND PHACOANAPHYLACTIC GLAUCOMA

Secondary open angle glaucoma may occur as a result of the obstruction of anterior chamber outflow channels by cells and particulate matter. When obstruction is due to intraocular blood or inflammatory cells associated with retained lens material, vitrectomy can be used to remove the blood or lens material and cure the glaucoma.

Hemolytic glaucoma

Vitreous hemorrhage may be complicated by hemolytic glaucoma. Macrophages filled with hemoglobin breakdown products and erythrocyte cellular debris mechanically obstruct the trabecular outflow channels, resulting in elevated intraocular pressure. This condition is seen most commonly in aphakic eyes; and, until the blood clears, the intraocular pressure may be difficult to control. When vitreous hemorrhage causes hemolytic glaucoma with uncontrollable intraocular pressure, vitrectomy can be used to clear the blood and cure the glaucoma. Hemolytic glaucoma is also occasionally seen after vitrectomy when loose blood remains in the eye. Usually the blood clears rapidly after vitrectomy and the intraocular pressure can be controlled with glaucoma therapy. If hemolytic glaucoma occurs after vitrectomy, however, and the intraocular pressure cannot be satisfactorily controlled, the remaining blood can be washed from the eye using a two-needle technique to provide infusion and suction through the peripheral clear cornea (in aphakic eyes).

Phacolytic and phacoanaphylactic glaucoma

Retained lens material after cataract surgery may elicit an inflammatory response resulting in secondary glaucoma caused by inflammatory cells obstructing the trabecular outflow cannels. Retained lens cortex is usually absorbed without complications, but cortical material may be phagocytosed by large macrophages which can obstruct the filtering trabeculum and cause phacolytic glaucoma. Retained nuclear material generally does not absorb spontaneously and often elicits a marked inflammatory response. The eye may become sensitized to lens protein and develop an intense granulomatous reaction involving the anterior uveal tract and surrounding the lens material (phacoanaphylactic endophthalmitis). Removal of retained cortical material is indicated if phacolytic glaucoma develops and the intraocular pressure cannot be satisfactorily controlled. Removal of nuclear material is often necessary to prevent loss of the eye due to the intense inflammatory reaction.

The pars plana vitrectomy technique provides a valuable method to remove lens material from the vitreous cavity. Cortical material is easily aspirated into the suction port. Nuclear material, however, may be sufficiently hard not to mold into the cutting port. In this situation we use suction to grasp the nucleus and bring it into the pupillary space, where it is mechanically crushed between the

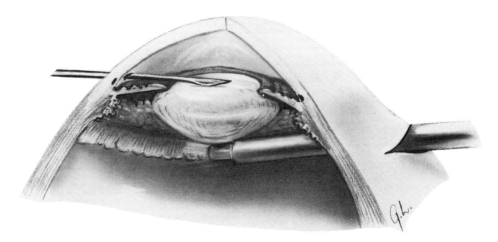

Fig. 9-18. A hard lens nucleus is supported in the pupillary space and mechanically crushed between the flat side of a knife blade and the vitrectomy instrument tip.

vitrectomy instrument and a knife introduced into the anterior chamber through peripheral clear cornea (Fig. 9-18). The lens fragments fall posteriorly and are retrieved with the vitrectomy instrument and further crushed. The smaller fragments are aspirated into the cutting port and removed.

We have successfully used this technique to treat phacolytic glaucoma caused by retained cortical material in the vitreous (Fig. 9-19). Also we have successfully removed a lens nucleus from the vitreous cavity associated with considerable local inflammation and secondary glaucoma (Fig. 9-20, A). In the latter case the procedure was lengthy because the hard nucleus had to be crushed by the two-instrument technique. Vision improved from 20/300 to 20/80 postoperatively, and the eye was quiet 6 months after surgery (Fig. 9-20, B), but mild corneal edema has persisted due to endothelial damage caused by the prolonged operation.

ENDOPHTHALMITIS

Endophthalmitis, especially after intraocular surgery, may rapidly produce a vitreous abscess. Bacteria proliferate in the vitreous and elicit a marked inflammatory response. This process often clears slowly despite intensive antibiotic and steroid therapy, and the eye may be destroyed by the inflammatory reaction despite successful elimination of the causative organism. Vitrectomy can be used to obtain biopsy material to identify the causative organism and to remove the necrotic cellular debris that excites further inflammatory cell infiltration; and it may lead to organization of the vitreous. Occasionally vitreous biopsy is necessary to differentiate between bacterial and mycotic endophthalmitis.

We have used vitrectomy, combined with postoperative systemic antibiotic therapy, to successfully treat four eyes with bacterial endophthalmitis and vitre-

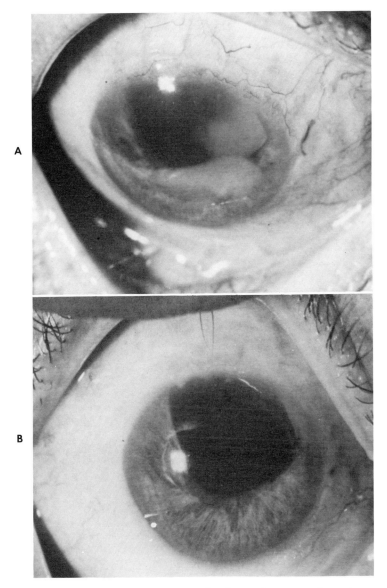

Fig. 9-19. A, Retained lens cortex in the anterior chamber and vitreous after extracapsular cataract extraction causing phacolytic glaucoma and uncontrollable intraocular pressure. **B,** Postoperative appearance 6 months after removal of the retained lens material by the pars plana vitrectomy technique. Vision is correctable to 20/20; intraocular pressure is normal.

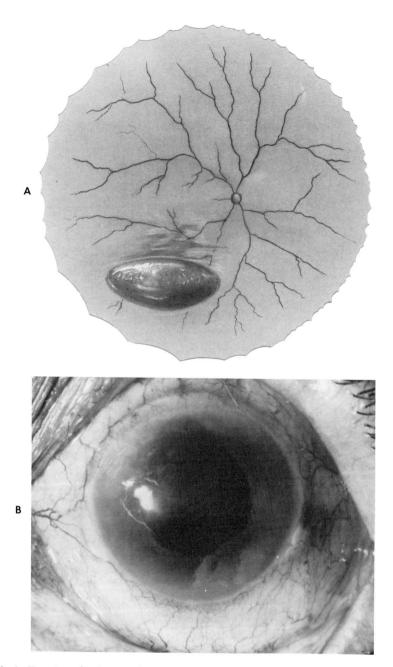

Fig. 9-20. A, Drawing of a lens nucleus in the inferior vitreous after an unplanned extracapsular cataract extraction which caused moderate inflammation and secondary glaucoma. **B,** Postoperative appearance 6 months after removal of the lens nucleus from the vitreous cavity by the pars plana vitrectomy technique. Though mild ciliary injection and central corneal edema persist, intraocular pressure is normal.

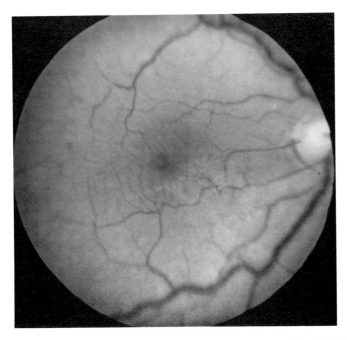

Fig. 9-21. Fundus appearance 7 days after vitrectomy for bacterial endophthalmitis with vitreous abscess. Six months after surgery, vision is correctable to 20/20.

ous abscess. In each case the inflammatory reaction cleared rapidly after vitrectomy, and vision improved (Fig. 9-21). Antibiotics were not placed in the vitreous cavity at the time of surgery. We do not know whether intracameral antibiotic doses, recommended for injection into the vitreous body, would be toxic to the retina in eyes with a fluid vitreous cavity. We reserve vitrectomy for eyes with significant vitreous abscess formation in which the inflammatory reaction is likely to result in loss of the eye despite intensive antibiotic therapy.

OTHER INDICATIONS

The pars plana vitrectomy technique can be used in other conditions when it is necessary to remove tissue or create intraocular structural alterations. We have used this technique to treat one eye with presumed nematode endophthalmitis in which a thick taut vitreous band extended between a white mass in the periphery of the fundus and the optic nerve. Vision in the eye was reduced to 20/100, and fluorescein angiography showed marked dilatation of and leakage from the capillaries on the optic nerve (Fig. 9-22, *A*). After the vitreous band was cut, vision improved to 20/25 and repeat fluorescein angiography showed less leakage from the small vessels on the nerve head (Fig. 9-22, *B* and *C*).

The role of vitreous surgery in the management of proliferative diabetic retinopathy is uncertain. At present we restrict vitrectomy to eyes blinded by nonresolving vitreous hemorrhage or recent traction detachment involving the macula; but we have been impressed by the observation that proliferative

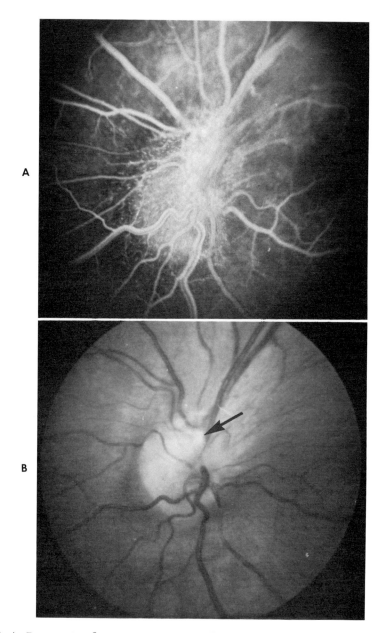

Fig. 9-22. A, Preoperative fluorescein angiogram of nematode endophthalmitis with vitreous traction on the optic nerve associated with marked dilatation and leakage from the capillary bed. **B,** Postoperative appearance after cutting of the vitreous band, relieving the traction on the optic nerve. The cut end of the band is indicated by the arrow.

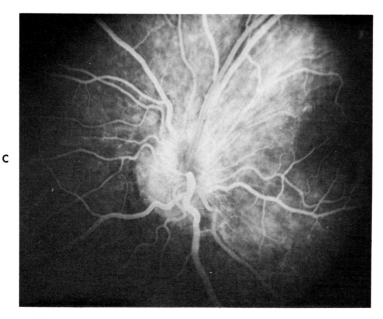

Fig. 9-22, cont'd. C, Fluorescein angiogram 6 months after cutting of the vitreous band. There is less dilatation and leakage from the capillaries on the optic nerve head.

retinopathy often remains quiescent after vitrectomy. It is possible that earlier vitrectomy might prevent some of the late complications by removing the vitreous scaffolding on which preretinal vessels grow and which can contract and cause retinal detachment. There are considerable operative risks associated with the vitrectomy procedure, however, and the role of vitrectomy earlier in the course of proliferative diabetic retinopathy should be explored only in a clinical trial designed to minimize the risks for the individual patient and yet provide meaningful data.

REFERENCES

1. Barr, C. C., Green, W. R., Payne, J. W., Knox, D. L., Jensen, A. D., and Thompson, R. L.: Intraocular reticulum-cell sarcoma: clincopathologic study of four cases and review of the literature, Survey Ophthalmol. 19:244, 1975.
2. Douvas, N. G.: The cataract Roto-Extractor, Trans. Am. Acad. Ophthalmol. Otolaryngol. 77:792, 1973.
3. Federman, J. L., Sarin, L. K., Annesley, W., Tasman, W., and McDonald, P. R.: Suction infusion tissue extractor (SITE). Presented at the meeting of the Retina Society, Montreal, September, 1974.
4. Iliff, C. E.: Treatment of the vitreous tug syndrome, Am. J. Ophthalmol. 62:856, 1966.
5. Jack, R. L., Hutton, W. L., and Machemer, R.: Ultrasonography and vitrectomy, Am. J. Ophthalmol. 78:265, 1974.
6. Kloeti, R.: Vitrektomie. 1, Ein neues Instrument fuer die hintere Vitrektomie, Graefe. Arch. Ophthalmol. 187:161, 1973.
7. Kreiger, A. E., Straatsma, B. R., Griffin, J. R., Storm, F. K., and Smiley, E. H.: A vitrectomy instrument in stereotaxic intraocular surgery, Am. J. Ophthalmol. 76:527, 1973.
8. L'Esperance, F. A., Jr., James, W. A., Jr., Hewson, T. A., and Fleischman, J. A.: A disposable vitreous cutter-aspirator with electronic vacuum control, Am. J. Ophthalmol. 79:674, 1975.
9. Machemer, R.: A new concept for vitreous surgery. II, Surgical technique and complications, Am. J. Ophthalmol. 74:1022, 1972.

10. Machemer, R.: A new concept for vitreous surgery. VI, Anesthesia and improvements in surgical technique, Arch. Ophthalmol. **92**:402, 1974.

11. Machemer, R.: A new concept for vitreous surgery. VII, Two-instrument techniques in pars plana vitrectomy, Arch. Ophthalmol. **92**:407, 1974.

12. Machemer, R.: Vitrectomy: a pars plana approach, New York, 1975, Grune & Stratton, Inc.

13. Machemer, R., Buettner, H., and Norton, E. W. D.: Vitrectomy: a pars plana approach, Trans. Am. Acad. Ophthalmol. Otolaryngol. **75**:813, 1971.

14. Machemer, R., and Norton, E. W. D.: A new concept for vitreous surgery. III, Indications and results, Am. J. Ophthalmol. **74**:1034, 1972.

15. Machemer, R., Parel, J. M., and Buettner, H.: A new concept for vitreous surgery. I, Instrumentation, Am. J. Ophthalmol. **73**:1, 1972.

16. Machemer, R., Parel, J. M., and Norton, E. W. D.: Vitrectomy: a pars plana approach. Technical improvements and further results, Trans. Am. Acad. Ophthalmol. Otolaryngol. **76**:462, 1972.

17. Michels, R. G.: Surgical management of selected non-magnetic intraocular foreign bodies, Arch. Ophthalmol. **93**:1003, 1975.

18. Michels, R. G., Knox, D. L., Erozan, Y. S., and Green, W. R.: Intraocular reticulum-cell sarcoma: diagnosis by pars plana vitrectomy, Arch. Ophthalmol. **93**:1331, 1975.

19. Michels, R. G., Machemer, R., and Müller-Jensen, K.: Vitreous surgery: history and current concepts, Ophthalmic Surg. **5**:13, 1974.

20. Norton, E. W. D.: Intraocular gas in the management of selected retinal detachments, Trans. Am. Acad. Ophthalmol. Otolaryngol. **77**:85, 1973.

21. Norton, E. W. D., Aaberg, T., Fung, W., and Curtin, V. T.: Giant retinal tears. I, Clinical management with intravitreal air, Am. J. Ophthalmol. **68**:1011, 1969.

22. Norton, E. W. D., and Machemer, R.: A new approach to the treatment of selected retinal detachments secondary to vitreous loss at cataract surgery, Am. J. Ophthalmol. **72**:705, 1971.

23. O'Malley, C., and Heintz, R. M.: Vitrectomy via the pars plana. A new instrument system, Trans. Pac. Coast Otoophthalmol. Soc. **53**:121, 1972.

24. Parel, J. M., Machemer, R., and Aumayr, W.: A new concept for vitreous surgery. IV, Improvements in instrumentation and illumination, Am. J. Ophthalmol. **77**:6, 1974.

25. Peyman, G. A., and Dodich, N. A.: Experimental vitrectomy: instrumentation and surgical technique, Arch. Ophthalmol. **86**:548, 1971.

26. Schepens, C. L.: Vitreous surgery: tissue removal. In Pruett, R. C., and Regan, D. J., editors: Retina Congress, New York, 1972, Appleton-Century-Crofts.

10

Pars plana vitrectomy in advanced diabetic retinopathy

Eighty consecutive cases performed with the Douvas Roto-Extractor

EDWARD OKUN

With the advent of photocoagulation, there have been many fewer cases of proliferative diabetic retinopathy reaching the advanced stages.[4,7,8] Nevertheless, until the basic cause of this occlusive vascular disease is elucidated, there will be eyes that are first detected in a stage too advanced to benefit from photocoagulation or there will be certain resistant forms of the disease, particularly those with neovascularization originating from the disc,[7] that go on to extensive intravitreal proliferation, organized vitreous hemorrhage, and/or traction retinal detachment with or without treatment. Pars plana vitrectomy has brought the first ray of hope to these previously "hopeless" cases.[2] Piecemeal removal of the opacified vitreous has benefitted these eyes in two ways: It has cleared the media, allowing focused light to strike the retina once again, and it has removed a source of traction to the proliferative membranes and the retina.

TECHNIQUE AND METHOD
Anesthesia

All patients are operated on under general anesthesia[3] with complete muscle paralysis and artificial respiration. Of particular value has been suctioning the stomach just prior to extubation. This maneuver has essentially eliminated any postoperative vomiting.

Equipment

The operating microscope is carefully checked and adjusted to be certain that the assistant's view is parfocal with the surgeon's and that the ranges of x-y movement and fine focus are within the limits desired for the case. The cutting port of the Roto-Extractor[1] is then examined to be certain that the cutting blade contacts the entire inner edge of the port as it rotates. All cutting is done with the 0.4 mm side cutting needle. If the lens is to be removed, the coring trephine is examined at its cutting tip to ensure that its edge is smooth and clean and that it rotates smoothly. The inflow and outflow tubing is cleared of air bubbles, and the spindle chamber is filled with irrigating solution.

Corneal epithelium

The corneal epithelium is usually removed at the beginning of the procedure if it appears to be loosely adherent to Bowman's membrane. This can be determined by gently rubbing a smooth forceps over the cornea to see whether the epithelium tends to move over Bowman's membrane. Nine times out of ten, the operator can remove the epithelium by grasping it near the center of the cornea with a serrated conjunctival forceps and tenting it upward away from Bowman's membrane. With one twisting maneuver the entire epithelium can be removed as a sheet with clean peripheral edges. If the epithelium is not removed at this stage, it will probably have to be cut away later since edematous epithelium greatly impairs visualization of the deeper structures.

Step-by-step

The entry sclerotomy is made by an incision in the inferior temporal quadrant just under the lateral rectus muscle, 4.5 mm posterior to and parallel with the limbus. If there is a peripheral membrane or retinal detachment in this quadrant, the site of entry is shifted to the superior temporal quadrant.

1. The conjunctiva is opened by a radial incision, and the leaves kept separated by two 4-0 silk fixation sutures placed through half-thickness sclera.
2. A 3 mm scratch incision is made with a Beaver blade, and the superficial vessels cauterized.
3. If a pars plana lensectomy is to be performed, the equator of the lens is entered via the sclerotomy site with a 1.7 mm sclerotome.
4. The end cutting trephine is used to fragment the lens nucleus and cortex by producing tunnels in the lens.
5. Once the lens has been thoroughly opacified by this "honeycombing" technique, the 0.4 mm side cutting needle is introduced and the nucleus and cortical material removed within the lens capsule.
6. The posterior capsule and the anterior vitreous are removed.
7. At this point the 0.4 mm side cutter is removed and the light pipe added.
8. The sclerotomy is enlarged with the 2.9 mm sclerotome making a sweeping motion through the vitreous base.
9. Utilizing a corneal forceps the surgeon grasps the posterior lip of the sclerotomy while the assistant grasps the anterior tip, both cooperating to spread the lips open. The adequacy of the opening should be judged at this time. If the opening appears too small, it is enlarged with the tip

of the sclerotome or the Vannas scissors, special care being taken to include the choroid in the opening. Too large an opening should be avoided since leakage around the vitrectomy instrument results in a less controlled vitrectomy.

10. The tip of the vitrectomy needle enters the sclerotomy easily, but the shoulder of the snugly fitting light pipe is pushed and rotated through the opening with difficulty.

11. Once the tip is through the sclera, there is a sudden loss of resistance and the movement of the instrument can be seen through the pupil—either indirectly, through movement of the vitreous, or directly, via a glimpse of the reflective metal itself.

12. The light pipe is turned on and the infusion fluid is allowed to reenter the eye, thus rebuilding the pressure up to normal.

13. The cutter is activated, and with gentle suction the vitreous around the instrument is removed—exposing the tip of the extractor.

14. Any vitreous trapped between the light pipe and the side cutting needle is freed by one of two motions: (a) gradually rotating the handle over 360° and back or (b) withdrawing the entire tip of the Roto-Extractor into the light pipe and then pushing the instrument out again until the tip and inflow ports are cleared. Gentle cutting and suction are maintained during each of these maneuvers.

15. From this point on, one never loses sight of the cutting port. A Goldmann contact lens adapted with an irrigating cannula is put on the cornea and kept in place through most of the remainder of the operation.

16. The vitreous is slowly and systematically extracted from the eye, moving gradually posteriorly until a hole is made in the posterior hyaloid. When the vitreous is opacified, this usually affords the first view of the retina. Until the retina is sighted, one must assume that it may be elevated and just under each opaque membrane being extracted.

17. Once the retina is sighted, more definite action can proceed—enlarging the hole in the membrane and uncovering more of the retina until fibro-vascular proliferative membranes are identified. These are usually easily recognized by their more grayish color and their attachments to the disc and retina.

18. Each membrane is freed from the vitreous; and when several such stalks are noted to be interconnected by bridges, the connections are severed—allowing each stalk to coil back on itself toward its site of origin on the retina or disc. The slight bleeding which may occur at this time is usually easily controlled by switching to the higher bottle (intraocular tamponade).

In the course of the vitrectomy for opacified vitreous hemorrhage, pockets of optically dense smokey-appearing fluid are opened and irrigated. This maneuver may completely obscure all vision for several minutes; but if gentle suction is maintained during this time, these pockets are gradually cleared.

Before the macular zone is inspected for membranes and potential visual function, attention is transferred again to the anterior capsule, under which some of the stirred up vitreous debris may have collected. The anterior capsule and residual cortical material are removed. The capsule may prove to be very resistant. It is best engaged with the cutting port open and cut with the oscillatory mode.

When the cutter is activated, a round hole is made in the capsule. This is repeated many times until a free edge is produced which can be enlarged to at least a 5 mm opening. To protect the corneal endothelium from the turbulent currents set up during the course of the vitrectomy the anterior capsule is best left until this stage of the procedure.

The anterior capsule may be very difficult to visualize at this time; but when the cutter is angled in various directions, the fiber-optic light defines the residual capsule adequately. Care must also be taken at this time to avoid inadvertent tears in the iris.

Since removal of the anterior capsule allows a much clearer view of the posterior pole, attention is once again focused on the macula. If posterior membranes are obscuring the macula, they may have to be removed. Sometimes a layer of blood appears trapped under a paramacular membrane. If the Roto-Extractor tip can be placed between the retina and the membrane with the cutting port directed toward the membrane and away from the retina, the membrane can be

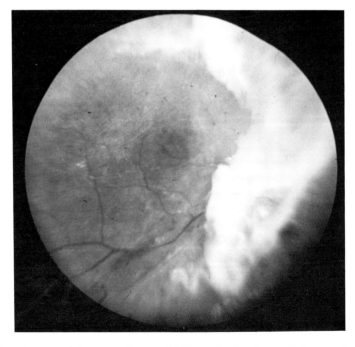

Fig. 10-1. Opening carved in a membrane which previously obscured the nasal part of the macula.

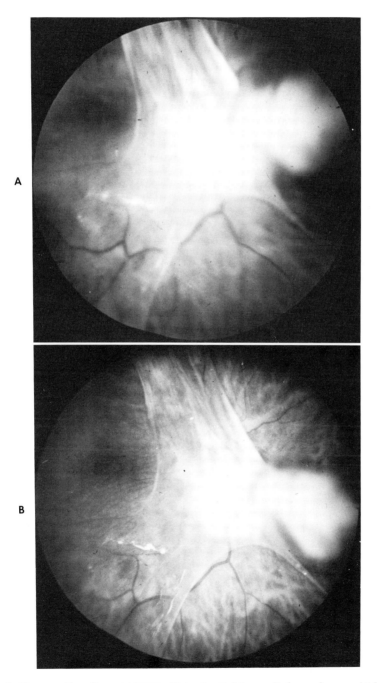

Fig. 10-2. A, Two months after vitrectomy. Note the lightly applied membrane which crosses the paramacular area. Visual acuity is 20/100. **B,** One year after vitrectomy. The membrane crossing the paramacular area has become thinner. Visual acuity is 20/80.

gradually lifted and removed utilizing gentle suction and the oscillatory mode for cutting. As long as the cutting port can be visualized directed away from the retina, there is little danger to the retina. Many posteriorly located membranes have been removed in this way (Fig. 10-1).

If the membrane is intimately adherent to the retina, I leave it. This has resulted in surprisingly good visual return in some instances. Certain of these membranes may still have to be removed by a second procedure before the operator can be certain that they are adversely affecting macular function. These membranes tend to become thinner as they are observed over the postoperative period (Fig. 10-2). Surprisingly few instances of either recurrent hemorrhage or subsequent macular visual loss have been observed in eyes where these tightly applied membranes were left in place.

At the end of the vitrectomy, there may still be oozing from the cut ends of the fibrovascular tissue. Certain of the more heavily vascularized stalks continue to hemorrhage postoperatively if not treated. For this purpose a two-pronged wet field diathermy coagulator[5] has been designed. A 1 mm Graefe knife is used to make a tract into the vitreous 4.5 mm behind the limbus in the superior nasal quadrent. The diathermy needle is placed through the tract and directed toward the leaking stalk. The Roto-Extractor continues to supply the light and irrigation as the two-pronged needle is placed in such a way that the stalk lies between

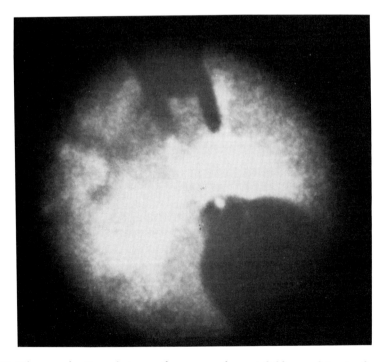

Fig. 10-3. Fibrovascular tissue between the prongs of a wet field coagulator in the process of being diathermized. Photograph taken through the operating microscope during surgery.

the prongs (Fig. 10-3). The current is then activated—resulting in immediate coagulation, shrinkage of the entrapped tissue, and complete cessation of the hemorrhage.

On one occasion this coagulation technique successfully closed a pumping arteriole.

When the vitreous has been cleared, all traction forces interrupted, and all significant bleeding controlled, it is time to terminate the procedure. With the instrument still in the eye, the operator inspects the fundus by indirect ophthal-moscopy to be certain no areas of significant traction or opacity have been overlooked and to check for retinal detachment or dialysis. If all checks out well, the infusion bottle is turned off and the intraocular pressure is allowed to fall. At this point it is wise to check once again for residual bleeding sites that may have to be coagulated. If there are none, the Roto-Extractor and light pipe and the diathermy (if used) are removed. The sclerotomy is closed with a running 9-0 monofilament nylon shoestring suture. The globe is reinflated with the irrigating solution and the conjunctiva closed with running 5-0 gut.

It may be well to emphasize that once the eye is entered with the Roto-Extractor and the light pipe is in place this instrument is not removed until the vitrectomy has been completed.

INDICATIONS

For purposes of consideration for vitrectomy, eyes with advanced diabetic retinopathy may be divided into three major categories:

1. Opacified vitreous secondary to long-standing vitreous hemorrhage
2. Traction retinal detachment secondary to fibrovascular proliferation and vitreous retraction
3. Fibrovascular proliferations with history of recurrent vitreous hemorrhage or evidence of spreading traction detachment

Once an organized vitreous hemorrhage turns grayish or greenish in color and shows definite membrane formation on ultrasound, it will probably take years to clear, if it ever clears. If no clearance has occurred over a one-year period and if potential vision in the affected eye will add substantially to the patient's vision, this eye becomes a candidate for vitrectomy. In instances of bilateral blindness, 6 to 9 months are enough time to wait for signs of clearing.

Traction retinal detachments usually occur in eyes with clear vitreous, and they tend to spread quite slowly. If the macula becomes detached or if the documented spreading pattern places the macula in imminent danger, something should be done. If anteroposterior traction forces can be clearly identified, with proliferative membranes connecting the retracted vitreous to the detached retina, these eyes may be candidates for vitrectomy combined with a scleral buckling procedure. If indentation alone appears to counteract the traction effects, however, or if retinal breaks are present, a scleral buckling procedure alone should be tried.

Fibrovascular proliferation into the vitreous usually precedes both the organized vitreous hemorrhage and the traction retinal detachment. If the proliferation is extensive and recurrent hemorrhages have been frequent and severe, or if the area of traction elevation of the retina is spreading, it may be possible to avoid a future inoperable retinal detachment or a long period of blindness secondary to vitreous hemorrhage by removing the vitreous and the fibrovascular proliferation at an earlier stage. The risk of the surgery in these instances must be weighed against the natural history of the eye so affected. This possible indication is under investigation. If the surgery can be performed without major short-term or long-term complications, this could prove to be the major indication for vitrectomy.

RESULTS

A review of 120 consecutive vitrectomies reveals that ninety (75%) were performed for advanced diabetic retinopathy. An analysis of the first eighty vitrectomies performed on diabetics shows the following indications: opacified vitreous, sixty eyes (75%), traction retinal detachments, thirteen eyes (16%), and retinitis proliferans, seven eyes (9%).

If visual improvement is used as a criterion for success, forty-two of sixty or 70% of the vitrectomies performed for opacified media were successful. Since essentially all the eyes had light-perception or hand-motion visual acuity to begin with, improved vision indicates visual acuity of count fingers or better. Table 10-1 shows a breakdown of final visual acuities in this group.

It is more difficult to establish parameters of success or failure in the eyes with traction retinal detachments or retinitis proliferans. Of the thirteen eyes operated on for traction retinal detachment, only three had slight visual improvement. The retina was completely reattached in only one, and two-thirds reattached in four. Frank failure occurred in seven. Scleral buckling procedures were employed in addition to the vitrectomy in six, and subsequent to the vitrectomy in two. At most, five of thirteen patients with traction retinal detachments benefitted from vitrectomy.

Vitrectomies performed on eyes with primary retinitis proliferans are equally difficult to evaluate, mainly because the follow-up is too short. One patient with an extremely vascular and extensive membrane covering and tightly applied to approximately eight disc areas of retina underwent vitrectomy to determine

Table 10-1. Final visual acuity after successful pars plana vitrectomy for opacified diabetic vitreous hemorrhage

Visual acuity	Number
20/20 - 20/30	5
20/40 - 20/60	6
20/70 - 20/100	6
20/200 - 20/400	17
Count fingers	8

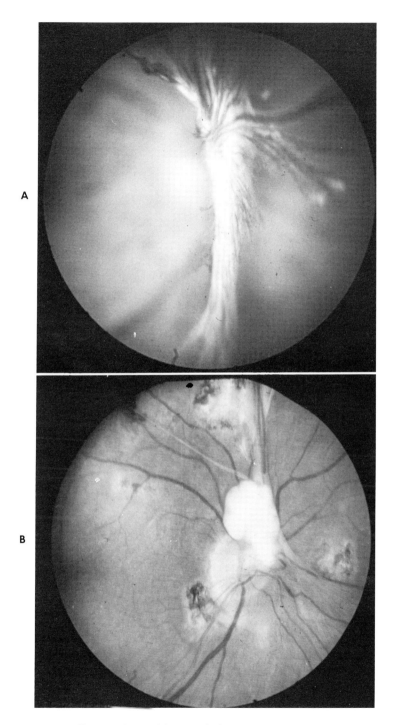

Fig. 10-4. **A,** Extensive fibrovascular proliferation before vitrectomy. Visual acuity is 20/25. **B,** One year after vitrectomy, 9 months after photocoagulation. Visual acuity is 20/30.

whether severing all vitreous adhesion to the membrane would be of any benefit. It was not. Another patient,[6] with a history of repeated severe vitreous hemorrhages, all of which had cleared (Fig. 10-4, *A*), underwent vitrectomy for extensive highly elevated neovascular membrane formation. This eye was subsequently photocoagulated, and at the one-year postvitrectomy examination the
vitrectomy appeared successful. The vitreous was crystal clear, visual acuity
was 20/30, and there had been no hemorrhages (Fig. 10-4, *B*). Three patients
have had various degrees of recurrent vitreous hemorrhage. One patient had a
dense hemorrhage during the third postoperative week, which did not clear
until the 6-month postoperative visit. At that visit visual acuity had improved to
20/400 compared to preoperative visual acuity of count fingers at 2 feet. A fibrovascular membrane that covered four disc areas of the posterior pole had been
greatly reduced (Fig. 10-5).

LENSECTOMY

Lensectomy was performed on thirty-six of the forty phakic eyes which were
operated on for organized vitreous hemorrhage. The lens was left in four eyes,
three of which have had recurrent vitreous hemorrhage. Twenty patients were
aphakic at the time of vitrectomy. It was unusual to find clear lenses in eyes with
long-standing vitreous hemorrhage.

Lenses were left intact in all seven patients with retinitis proliferans, and removed by pars plana lensectomy in only four of the thirteen patients with traction
retinal detachment. In one of these patients, a minimal cataract matured in 4
weeks. All other lenses appear not to have been affected by the procedure.

COMPLICATIONS

The major complications of pars plana vitrectomy in advanced diabetic
retinopathy are rubeosis iridis and retinal detachment. Transient elevation of
intraocular pressure and corneal edema are seen in the early postoperative period; but unless rubeosis iridis sets in, permanent glaucoma and corneal degeneration are rare.

Rubeosis iridis was observed postoperatively in eighteen of the first eighty
vitrectomies (23%). In seven of these eyes, rubeosis had been noted preoperatively. Other eyes with minimal preoperative involvement may have been overlooked since rubeosis iridis was not appreciated as a major complication until
recently. Ten of the eighteen eyes affected with rubeosis harbored hopelessly
detached retinas, four being operated on primarily for the retinal detachment.
Of the remaining eight, two appeared to have lost vision primarily because of
the hemorrhagic glaucoma. The other six eyes with rubeosis have continued to
function well, their pressures being controlled either medically or with the aid
of cyclocryotherapy (five cases). Last recorded visual acuities of these six eyes
were 20/20, 20/60, 20/100, 20/200, and finger counting at 3 feet.

It is of interest that when this group of advanced diabetics is divided into
eyes that were aphakic preoperatively and eyes that had either a combined len-

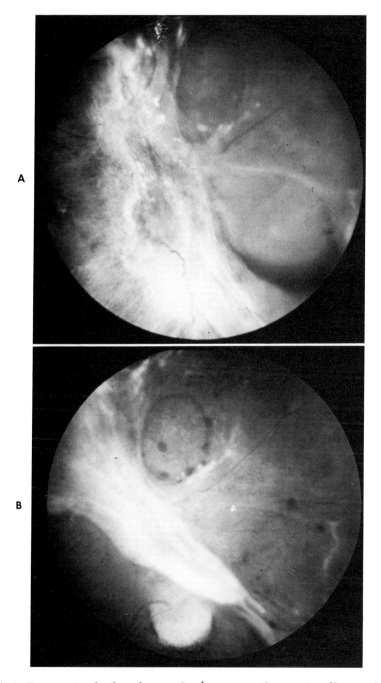

Fig. 10-5. A, Preoperative fundus photograph of an eye with extensive fibrovascular membrane formation obscuring the disc. Visual acuity is count fingers at 2 feet. **B,** Six months after vitrectomy. Visual acuity is 20/400.

sectomy-vitrectomy or a vitrectomy with the lens left in the incidence of rubeosis appears to be much less in the aphakic eyes. Only one of eighteen aphakic patients developed rubeosis after vitrectomy (excluding two aphakes known to have had rubeosis prior to vitrectomy), as compared to eight of thirty-three patients undergoing combined lensectomy vitrectomy (excluding five eyes known to have had rubeosis preoperatively).

Retinal detachment can occur any time during the postoperative period, but usually during the first month. In two eyes a retinal detachment associated with dialysis was discovered on the operating table. In another two cases the detachment was detected during the first 5 postoperative days. The remaining five occurred during the first month, for a total nine out of eighty (11%). Six of the nine were successfully repaired. One unsuccessfully operated retinal detachment occurred in the first vitrectomy performed and was complicated by an inadequate removal of opaque vitreous and the development of massive preretinal fibrosis. The other two occurred in patients too ill to undergo further surgery. Both these patients subsequently expired. The six patients undergoing successful scleral buckling procedures had visual acuities of 20/40, 20/100, 20/400 + 2, count fingers at 2 feet, and hand motion. The hand-motion patient underwent vitrectomy for fibrovascular proliferative membranes and repeated vitreous hemorrhage. Visual acuity of 20/40 was achieved after the scleral buckling procedure, but a recurrent vitreous hemorrhage subsequently reduced visual acuity to hand motion only.

There have been only two permanent corneal problems other than those associated with rubeosis iridis. The first occurred in a patient who had had a history of recurrent corneal erosion sixteen years earlier and in whom the condition was reactivated. She has worn a soft contact lens intermittently since the second postoperative week. The cornea became vascularized, but the vessels retreated when the lens was removed. The other patient with a residual corneal problem had an acute episode of severe eye pain, swelling, corneal infiltration, and hypopion after soft contact lens wear during the third postoperative week. This condition was treated like an endophthalmitis despite a negative anterior chamber culture. The eye has gradually cleared but the cornea has remained minimally edematous. Visual acuity is 20/400.

Recurrent vitreous hemorrhage has been a complication only in cases of retinitis proliferans with actively growing neovascular membranes and in those few cases of organized vitreous hemorrhage in which the lenses were not removed.

COMMENTS

Pars plana vitrectomy combined with lensectomy is a very effective procedure in most cases of long-standing vitreous hemorrhage. Results are less gratifying in cases of traction retinal detachment. It is possible to perform vitrectomy in eyes with fibrovascular proliferation before traction retinal detachment or massive vitreous hemorrhage occurs. The major early problem appears to have been recurrent postoperative hemorrhage. It is too soon after the routine use of underwater diathermy on these actively growing membranes to say whether vitrectomy will solve the problem. If the answer proves to be positive, the no. 1 indication for vitrectomy may be the presence of actively growing or contracting intravitreal fibrovascular proliferation.

Lens extraction of and by itself seems to excite rubeosis iridis in certain diabetic eyes. The aphakic eyes which came to vitrectomy in our series had probably already proved that they could resist this stimulus, whereas those undergoing combined lensectomy vitrectomy were not preselected. Subjecting vitrectomy candidates to routine cataract surgery 2 months prior to planed vitrectomy may aid materially in the selection of eyes capable of withstanding surgery without the development of rubeosis. Eyes which do develop rubeosis may be treated by cyclocryotherapy prior to vitrectomy, or rejected for vitrectomy if the rubeosis cannot be controlled.

Retinal detachment occurs after the production of either a dialysis or a retinal hole. The dialysis is probably related to extensive tugging or pushing at the vitreous base. The right-angle shoulder at the junction of the needle and the light pipe is the weak point in the design of the internal light source. The vitreous base must be widely opened with the knife prior to the introduction of the light pipe, and care must be taken to free vitreous fibrils from the light pipe prior to pushing the instrument toward the other side of the eye. The cutting efficiency of the needle should be tested repeatedly by turning off suction and cutting all vitreous free from the cutting port. If the needle is not cutting well, vitreous should be expelled or regurgitated from the cutting port and a new cutting needle used. Retinal tears can be produced by inefficient cutting action, particularly on proliferative membranes which are close to the retina. The oscillatory mode should be used in this location as insurance against winding a membrane instead of cutting it cleanly.

For the purpose of clearing opacified vitreous, a lensectomy should probably be performed in conjunction with the vitrectomy. A more complete vitrectomy can be performed with the lens removed, and residual or small recurrent hemorrhages seem to clear more rapidly in aphakic eyes.

SUMMARY

Forty-two of sixty eyes (70%) undergoing vitrectomy or lensectomy—vitrectomy for opacified vitreous hemorrhage in advanced diabetic retinopathy had improved visual acuity. Five of thirteen eyes (38%) with traction retinal detachments appeared to have benefitted from vitrectomy. Three of seven patients who had vitrectomy for retinitis proliferans appeared to have benefitted. Recurrent vitreous hemorrhage has been a problem in this last group.

Rubeosis iridis and retinal detachment have been the major complications noted in our series of eighty consecutive vitrectomies performed on eyes with advanced diabetic retinopathy.

EDITOR'S NOTE

Dr. Okun's introduction of the use of a wet field diathermy coagulator is highly significant since vitrectomy done without closure of large-caliber neovascular fronds at surgery often results in recurrent vitreous hemorrhage. Perhaps this technique will offer a means of closing these vessels, as beautifully illustrated in his example of a juvenile diabetic with extensive disc neovascularization before and after vitrectomy (Fig. 10-3). The entire subject of early vitrectomy in cases of proliferative diabetic retinopathy with or without opacified vitreous is the subject of a presently ongoing N.I.H. study.

REFERENCES

1. Douvas, N. G.: The cataract Roto-Extractor (a preliminary report), Trans. Am. Acad. Ophthalmol. Otolaryngol. **77**:792, 1973.
2. Machemer, R., Buettner, H., Norton, E. W. D., and Parel, J. M.: Vitrectomy: a pars plana approach, Trans. Am. Acad. Ophthalmol. Otolaryngol. **75**:813, 1971.
3. Meyers, E. F., and Wilson, S.: Vitrectomy—a new challenge for the anesthesiologist, Anesth. Analg. **54**:(1)58, 1975.
4. Okun, E.: The effectiveness of photocoagulation in the therapy of proliferative diabetic retinopathy (PDR) (a controlled study in 50 patients), Trans. Am. Acad. Ophthalmol. Otolaryngol. **72**:246, 1968.
5. Okun, E.: A two-pronged intravitreal wet-field coagulator. (In preparation.)
6. Okun, E., and Burgess, D. B.: Pars plana lensectomy and vitrectomy with the Douvas Roto-Extractor in diabetic retinopathy. Presented at the Symposium on Vitreous Surgery, San Francisco, March, 1974. (In press).
7. Okun, E., and Cibis, P. A.: The role of photocoagulation in the therapy of proliferative diabetic retinopathy, Arch. Ophthalmol. **75**:337, 1966.
8. Wetzig, P. C., and Jepson, C. N.: Treatment of diabetic retinopathy by light coagulation, Am. J. Ophthalmol. **62**:459, 1966.

11

Clinical experiences with the vitrophage

GHOLAM A. PEYMAN
FELIPE U. HUAMONTE
MORTON F. GOLDBERG

We have used our disposable instrument, the vitrophage,[1-4] and accessory instruments in over 100 pars plana vitrectomies. This report describes our instrumentation, techniques, and results of the first 100 vitrectomies.

INSTRUMENTATION
Vitrophage

The cutting action of the vitrophage is achieved by linear oscillation of the inner tube against an opening in the distal portion of the outer tube (Fig. 11-1). A space between the inner and outer tubes allows fluid infusion. The vitrophage is equipped with a fiber-optic illumination system for visualization inside the eye.

Lens fragmenter

The vitrophage is adapted as a lens fragmenter for pars plana lensectomy by shortening the distal end so the inner tube will protrude during oscillation (Fig. 11-2). This oscillation of the inner tube fragments the lens cortex and nucleus. The emulsified lens is then easily removed with the vitrophage.

Intraocular diathermy probe

The intraocular diathermy probe (Fig. 11-3) is used for coagulation of bleeding intravitreal vessels. Only twice in 160 vitrectomies has it been needed to coagulate the cut end of an intravitreal stalk.

We thank Jane Lantz for editorial assistance and Robert Parshall for medical illustrations. This investigation was supported in part by Public Health Service grant 1107-03 and by the Illinois Lions Club.

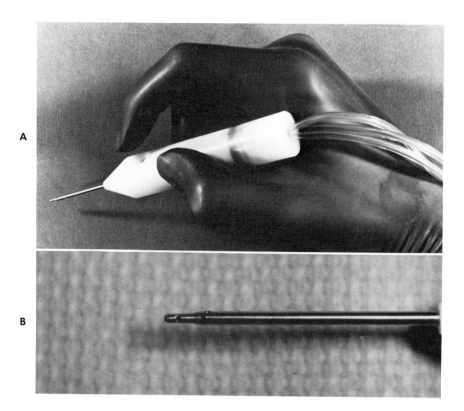

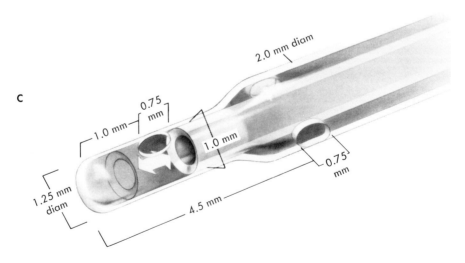

Fig. 11-1. The vitrophage. **A,** Note its dimension while in the operator's hand. The index finger points to the orifice for regulation of suction. **B,** Tip. **C,** Schematic diagram with dimensions. The cutting action is oscillatory and guillotine-like.

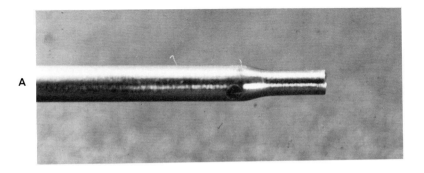

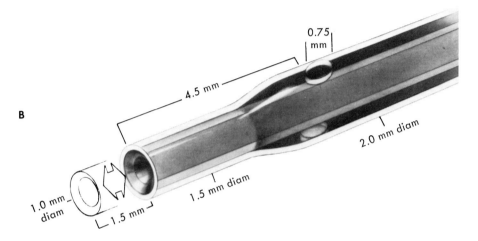

Fig. 11-2. A, Lens fragmenter tip. **B,** Schematic diagram with dimensions. Note the outward pulsation of the inner tube.

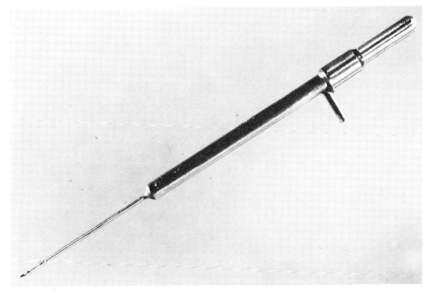

Fig. 11-3. Intraocular diathermy probe. Except for its tip, the probe is completely insulated. Infusion can be performed through the needle.

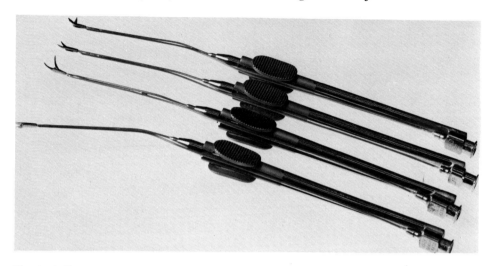

Fig. 11-4. Vitreous scissors and forceps. Note that the blades are bent away from the shaft to provide better visualization and a different angle of cutting.

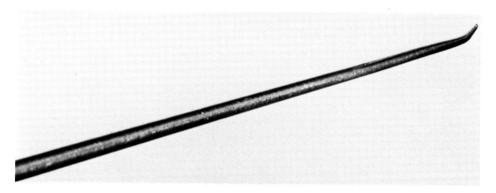

Fig. 11-5. Hook for dissection of preretinal membranes.

Vitreous scissors, forceps, and hook

Vitreous scissors, forceps, and hooks (Figs. 11-4 and 11-5) are used to dissect and remove preretinal membranes and intravitreal foreign bodies. A small tube permits infusion inside the eye during the operation.

TECHNIQUE

With some modifications, our technique for pars plana vitrectomy and lensectomy is similar to techniques described by other authors.

1. A 4 mm sclerotomy is performed parallel with and 4.5 mm behind the limbus in the temporal inferior or superior part of the globe.
2. The choroid is diathermized, and a 5-0 Dacron suture is applied to the scleral lips.
3. A no. 52S Beaver knife penetrates the eye to allow vitrophage insertion.

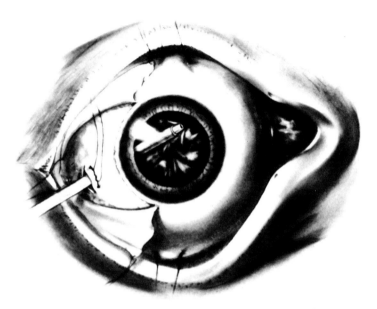

Fig. 11-6. Insertion of the lens fragmenter inside the lens for fragmentation of the lens nucleus and cortex.

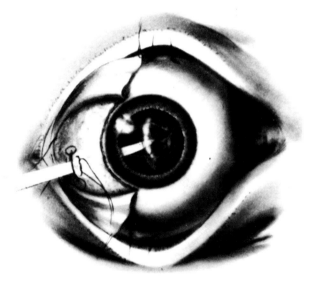

Fig. 11-7. When the Beaver knife cannot puncture the lens, the lens is too hard to be removed through the pars plana.

    If a lensectomy is needed because of cataract, the lens fragmenter is inserted along the knife track to emulsify the lens (Fig. 11-6).

4. The vitrophage cuts and removes the lens (technique 1). Vitrectomy always follows lens removal.

5. If the Beaver knife does not penetrate the lens (Fig. 11-7) and the lens dislocates, it is too hard to remove by this technique. Therefore the

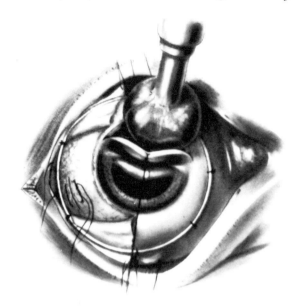

Fig. 11-8. Lens extraction through the clear cornea. Vitrectomy can be performed either immediately after closure of the cornea or at a later date.

sclerotomy is temporarily closed and a routine cataract extraction is performed through a clear corneal incision (technique 2) (Fig. 11-8).
6. The incision is closed by a continuous 9-0 nylon suture. Vitrectomy through the pars plana under the microscope and Goldmann contact lens follows lens extraction by this technique as well.

RESULTS

One hundred eyes of ninety-eight patients have been operated on because of vitreous opacities. Table 11-1[5] indicates the classification of postoperative improvement in visual acuity.

Diabetic vitreous hemorrhage

Group 1: Diabetic retinopathy with fibrovascular proliferation. Twenty-eight eyes had proliferative diabetic retinopathy detected either before or after the vitrectomy. Postoperative vision improved in twenty-three eyes (3+ in seven eyes, 2+ in ten eyes, and 1+ in six eyes), with an overall improvement of 82%.

COMPLICATIONS. In seven eyes minimal bleeding was encountered—from the iris, from a fibrovascular stalk at the disc, or from fibrovascular stalks outside the disc. The bleeding stopped either spontaneously or after the intraocular pressure was increased.

Postoperatively six eyes rebled, but the origin of the bleeding was undetectable. Only two eyes required subsequent vitreous lavage. Increase of intraocular pressure was noticed in eight eyes. In four eyes the elevation of intraocular

Table 11-1. Classification of visual improvement after vitrectomy*

	1+	2+	3+
Level I Light perception Hand motion Counting fingers 20/400	↓		
Level II 20/400 to 20/100	↓	↓	
Level III 20/100 to 20/20	↓	↓	↓

Code: *1+*, Improvement within any level.
 2+, Improvement to the next better level.
 3+, Improvement from level I to level III.

*From Peyman, G. A., Huamonte, F. U., and Goldberg, M. F.: One hundred consecutive pars plana vitrectomies with the vitrophage, Am. J. Ophthalmol. (In press.)

pressure was transient. Four eyes had glaucoma caused by blood products in the anterior chamber; these were controlled with acetazolamide.

Group 2: Proliferative diabetic retinopathy with tractional retinal detachment and vitreous hemorrhage. Twenty-four eyes were operated on in this group. The postoperative visual acuity was improved in fourteen eyes (3+ in one eye, 2+ in six eyes, and 1+ in seven eyes), with an overall improvement of 58%. In six eyes (25%) vision remained unchanged, and in four eyes (17%) it was worse. The follow-up ranged from 5 to 14 months, with a mean of 9 months.

COMPLICATIONS. Minimal hemorrhage occurred in four eyes—one from an iris vessel and three from undetected sites. Glaucoma was encountered in three eyes that developed rubeosis iridis. Transient corneal edema was seen in one eye. A questionable iatrogenic lens opacity was observed in one eye, although the postoperative visual acuity was 20/200 with a follow-up of 10 months and no progression of the opacity. In one eye an oval break, detected 1 month after vitrectomy in an area adjacent to localized tractional retinal detachment, remained stable with no increase of the detachment (6-month follow-up).

Nondiabetic vitreous hemorrhage

Twenty-eight eyes are included in the nondiabetic vitreous hemorrhage category.

Group 3: Trauma. In our series we had eight eyes with vitreous hemorrhage secondary to traumatic injury; four were contusional and four were penetrating injuries. Seven of the eight eyes had traumatic cataract. Postoperative visual acuity improved in four eyes (3+ in one eye, 2+ in one eye, 1+ in two). In the remaining four eyes visual acuity did not change. There were no operative complications in this group of eyes, and the postoperative course was uneventful.

Group 4: Central or branch vein occlusion. One eye had branch vein occlusion and two eyes had central vein occlusion causing vitreous hemorrhage of several years' duration. Postoperative vision improved in all three eyes (3+ in one eye and 1+ in the remaining two eyes). There were no surgical or postoperative complications. One eye developed transient elevation of the intraocular pressure that resolved in 1 week.

Group 5: Sickle cell retinopathy. Postoperative visual acuity initially improved in these two eyes (3+ and 1+). After we compiled the data, one patient had a repeat vitreous hemorrhage and elevation of intraocular pressure—resulting in no light perception.

Group 6: Vasculitis, systemic hypertension, and unknown etiology. Postoperative vision improved in three eyes (3+ in two eyes and 1+ in one eye) and was worse in two eyes.

Group 7: Retinal detachment with vitreous hemorrhage, membranes, or bands. The postoperative vision was improved in three eyes (2+ in two eyes and 1+ in one eye), remained unchanged in two, and was worse in one eye.

Group 8: Miscellaneous. In one eye with an intraocular nonmagnetic foreign body, the vision postoperatively improved to 20/20 but subsequently was reduced to 20/600 because of the development of macular pucker. Silicone oil was removed from the vitreous cavity of one eye; the vision did not improve postoperatively. One patient developed a fungal endophthalmitis *(Candida albicans)* after perforating injury. The vision improved after vitrectomy from light perception to 20/300. One patient had unplanned extracapsular cataract extraction with subsequently dislocated lens. Visual acuity had improved from a preoperative level of hand motion to 20/300 postoperatively.

Anterior segment opacities

Group 9: Secondary membranes after surgical trauma or perforating traumatic eye injuries (anterior segment reconstruction). Among eighteen eyes, postoperative visual acuity was improved in sixteen (3+ in one eye, 2+ in ten eyes, and 1+ in five eyes), with an overall improvement of 89% in this group. Vision remained unchanged in two (11%).

Group 10: Miscellaneous complications after cataract extraction. In one eye with vitreous adhesion to the cornea, vision after vitrectomy was improved to 20/60 after 6 months. Another patient who suffered epithelial downgrowth underwent anterior vitrectomy and iridectomy in addition to transcorneal cryocoagulation while air was injected into the anterior chamber. Postoperative vision was not improved.

DISCUSSION

The vitrophage can be set up for use quickly and easily. Since the cutting tip is air driven, there are no electrical connections in the vitrophage—thereby eliminating shock hazard. A trained assistant is not necessary since all aspects of the surgical procedure are under the control of the surgeon.

No retinal dialysis was observed at the end of the surgical procedures or during the follow-up period, even (as in the patient with sickle cell retinopathy) when the vitreous base was attacked. In addition, only one rhegmatogenous retinal detachment developed postoperatively.

Our cases fell into clearly divided groups:

One category included cases that allowed removal of opacities or cutting of bands or membranes with the vitrophage in the anterior part of the eye. The best visual results after vitrectomy were achieved in these patients. The use of the vitrophage in this group of patients produced results that were superior to the results achieved by older techniques—e.g., membranectomies or capsulectomies.

A second category included cases that required much manipulation, some of it close to the retina, to remove opacities, bands, or membranes in the deep vitreous. The reduced visual acuity in these patients was due mostly to preexistent macular damage resulting from vascular occlusions that were evident on fluorescein angiography.[6] The worst results occurred in diabetic patients with traction retinal detachment. These patients had localized or total retinal detachment often involving the macular area, which accounted for reduced visual acuity. We also had poor results in reattaching retinas in the presence of preretinal organization. We believe, however, that combined scleral buckling, vitrectomy, and gas injection offer the best hope of retinal reattachment in these cases.

Cases requiring removal of the lens deserve separate mention. The lens fragmenter and vitrophage worked well in breaking up lenses with moderate (1+ to 2+) nuclear sclerosis. We found that those nuclei that resisted penetration by the no. 52S blade were difficult to remove; consequently we use this inpenetrability as an indication to remove the lens through a 150° cataract incision at the corneoscleral limbus. Vitrectomy via the pars plana was continued after the corneal wound was sutured closed.[4]

The results of vitrectomy with the vitrophage, which depend in large measure on the status of the patient's retina and retinal vessels, have been encouraging. In eyes with posterior segment opacities, visual acuity was improved in 68%, unchanged in 20%, and worse in 12%. Eyes with anterior segment opacities had improved visual acuity in 85%; visual acuity was the same in 15%.

REFERENCES

1. Peyman, G. A., Daily, M. J., and Ericson, E. S.: Experimental vitrectomy, new technical aspects, Am. J. Ophthalmol. **75**:774, 1973.
2. Peyman, G. A., and Dodich, N. A.: Experiment vitrectomy, instrumentation and surgical technique, Arch. Ophthalmol. **86**:548, 1971.
3. Peyman, G. A., and Huamonte, F. U.: The vitrophage, a disposable vitrectomy instrument, Can. J. Ophthalmol. (In press.)
4. Peyman, G. A., Huamonte, F. U., and Goldberg, M. F.: Management of cataract in patients undergoing vitrectomy, Am. J. Ophthalmol. (In press.)
5. Peyman, G. A., Huamonte, F. U., and Goldberg, M. F.: One hundred consecutive pars plana vitrectomies with the vitrophage, Am. J. Ophthalmol. (In press.)
6. Peyman, G. A., Huamonte, F. U., Loketz, A., and Goldberg, M. F.: Fluorescein angiography of the fundus after pars plana vitrectomy, Can. J. Ophthalmol. (In press.)

12

Role of vitrectomy in trauma

D. JACKSON COLEMAN

Traumatic vitreous hemorrhage may result from contusion injury, lacerating injury, or retained reactive foreign body. The unique character of each traumatic injury, the individual status of the vitreous (i.e., formed or fluid vitreous), the time lapse since injury, and the resultant degree of inflammation all contribute to the complexity of planning surgical intervention.

Once vitreous involvement after ocular trauma has been determined, the preoperative selection of patients suitable for vitrectomy, the choice of procedure, and the proper timing of the surgery are the prime concerns of the surgeon. Complete assessment of vitreous damage includes evaluation of associated structures since the status of the retina, lens, ciliary body, anterior chamber, choroid and sclera influences the eventual recovery of vitreous clarity.

The vitreous would appear to be a useful but nonessential structure for adequate visual function, provided clarity of the space is maintained. After injury, however, this structure serves as a scaffold for fibroplastic changes that not only result in opacity but also permit the development of traction on the retina, particularly at the macula. Obviously in many injuries opacification is immediate and adequate visualization of the fundus by optical means is unobtainable. With ultrasonic evaluation a critical insight into the extent of the injury can be obtained and proper surgical management can be initiated.

In the evaluation of any traumatized eye, whether acute and untreated or on referral, after primary surgical closure has been performed, the prime question is whether surgical intervention is beneficial and, if so, what type of surgery is best. The new techniques afforded by vitreous suction and cutting instruments[6,7] allow us a means of intervention far more delicate and definitive than previous methods and thus require a reexamination of conventional surgical management of traumatized eyes.

Although the general rule that the least vitreous manipulation is best may still apply, there are many situations previously "inoperable" and conservatively followed to phthisis that may be benefited by early and often extensive vitrectomy.

Previous studies[5] have indicated that the following severe traumatic ocular changes are indications for vitrectomy:

1. Rupture of the lens capsule with subsequent dispersion of lens material into the vitreous
2. Massive hemorrhagic change in conjunction with ciliary body laceration or posterior globe perforation
3. Retinal detachment after traumatic vitreous hemorrhage
4. A retained reactive intraocular foreign body

These almost invariably result in permanent visual loss and often loss of the globe itself.

Although experience is not yet sufficiently extensive to establish absolute criteria, the progressive nature of hemorrhagic and inflammatory changes strongly militate for early surgical intervention (i.e., within 48 hours). If early intervention cannot be initiated, as is often the case, and the absence of a retained reactive foreign body or retinal detachment is ascertained, then a further delay of approximately 3 to 4 weeks may be tolerated and even preferable until the acute vitreous inflammatory stage has subsided. In general, surgery should be planned within 3 months in these types of trauma.

TRAUMATIC LENS RUPTURE

Injury to the lens resulting in rupture of the posterior capsule and mixture of lens material into the vitreous (Fig. 12-1) will produce an opacification of the

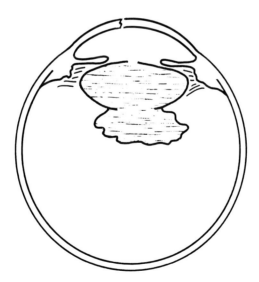

Fig. 12-1. Traumatic rupture of the posterior lens capsule with mixture of the lens material into the anterior vitreous, producing an opacification which requires lensectomy and vitrectomy.

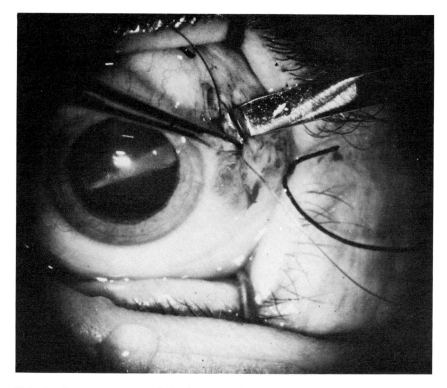

Fig. 12-2. A sclerotome incision of the lens capsule at the equator is made through a pars plana incision 4 mm from the limbus.

vitreous which prevents adequate visualization of the fundus. A severe vitritis often follows such an injury; and in our experience vitreous reaction has been more pronounced in young individuals with solid vitreous than in older individuals in whom the vitreous assumes a more fluid configuration. These inflammatory changes render the globe more susceptible to hemorrhage during surgery as well as produce a vitreous body with a dense rubbery consistency that is difficult to both cut and aspirate surgically. Vitrectomy at the earliest possible opportunity is thus recommended.

A routine incision (Fig. 12-2) is made through the pars plana parallel to the limbus at a distance of 4 mm. The pars plana incision is preferable to an open sky technique, since it minimizes trauma to an already damaged globe and provides maximum access to the plane of the ruptured lens. I prefer to use the phacoemulsifier (Fig. 12-3) to remove any lens material that may remain with the damaged capsule, but vitrectomy instruments are usually adequate. When the interior of the lens has been completely cleared, the vitrectomy instrument is introduced into the eye through the same incision site (Fig. 12-4) and capsule remnants and mixed lens and vitreous are then removed. If the remainder of the vitreous compartment is generally clear and fibroplastic activity or blood does not obscure the posterior pole, total vitrectomy is not usually required. In

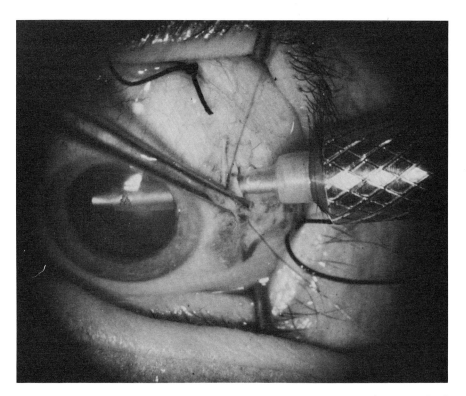

Fig. 12-3. The phacoemulsifier is introduced through a pars plana incision into the lens equator for removal of the lens material.

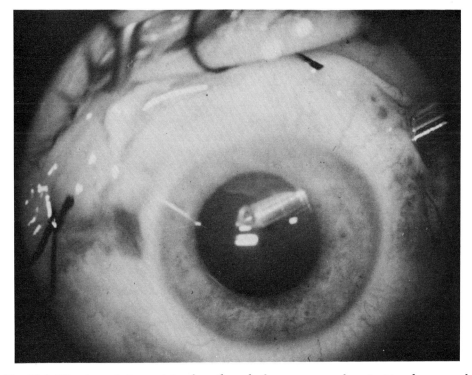

Fig. 12-4. Vitrectomy instrument in place through the same pars plana incision for removal of the lens capsule and subsequent vitrectomy.

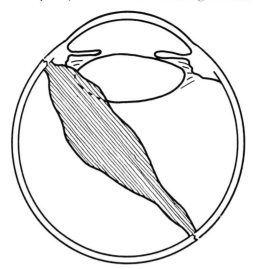

Fig. 12-5. Through-and-through laceration with opacification of the vitreous requiring vitrectomy and a prophylactic retinal detachment procedure.

the presence of hemorrhage or fibroplasia, however, aspiration of the vitreous, avoiding the area of the vitreous base, is then completed.

MASSIVE VITREOUS HEMORRHAGE WITH CILIARY BODY LACERATIONS OR POSTERIOR GLOBE PERFORATIONS

Ciliary body lacerations or posterior globe perforations (Fig. 12-5) accompanied by massive vitreous hemorrhage produce such profound intraocular changes that a poor prognosis is generally to be expected. Although certain of these globes may survive, only a small percentage are likely to maintain visual function. Formation of fibroplastic traction membranes along the path of vitreous disruption will contract with time, producing retinal detachment and/or ciliary body disinsertion. Early debridement of the vitreous planes and attachments not only allows more adequate visualization and repair of the wound but may prevent the membrane traction syndrome.

The surgical procedure in these eyes, with lens intact, is an incision 4.5 mm from the limbus temporally with subsequent instrumented removal of the anterior vitreous. A fiber-optic light source[8] is essential, for the anterior hyaloid may obscure visualization of the instrument tip. Damage to the lens capsule may be avoided by placement of the instrument tip 1 to 2 mm posterior to the lens capsule. This position may be gauged by the light flare at the tip of the fiber-optic. At this distance the opaque anterior vitreous can be suctioned backward to the instrument. The remainder of the total vitrectomy can then proceed in the conventional manner since visualization of the tip has been achieved by first clearing the retrolental space.

In certain scleral lacerations additional trauma to the globe may be avoided by introducing the instrument into the globe through the wound site. Exceptional care must be taken to avoid aspirating the ciliary body or retina when

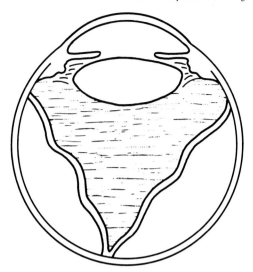

Fig. 12-6. Posttraumatic vitreous hemorrhage in conjunction with total retinal detachment requiring vitrectomy and a retinal detachment procedure.

the wound site is used thus. Unless good visualization can be obtained of this area through the cornea, a final debridement of the inner lips of the wound may still require a separate pars plana incision.

Vitreous membranes leading to a posterior perforation site form rapidly after injury and should be assiduously removed. The preoperative ultrasonic localization of the wound site may be instrumental in directing the posterior vitrectomy.

VITREOUS HEMORRHAGE WITH RETINAL DETACHMENT

Because a significant portion of vitritis and uveitis and consequent massive periretinal proliferation are related to the retinal detachment, ultrasonic demonstration of detachment in the presence of a traumatic vitreous hemorrhage (Fig. 12-6) is a strong indication for immediate vitrectomy.

The surgical approach is similar to that described for dense vitreous hemorrhage. When vitreous hemorrhage has been present for several weeks, inflammatory changes may produce a disinsertion of the retina at the ora, pulling the edges of the retina to the region of the iris root. Extreme care should therefore be exercised in aspirating opaque vitreous from this region to avoid inadvertent retinectomy. It is usually advisable first to identify the central retina and then to carefully aspirate vitreous forward along the retina until the area of peripheral retina can be identified.

Our present surgical procedure is to preplace a silicone band about the eye before the pars plana incision is made so that after vitrectomy, the tying of the band and completion of surgery are of relatively short duration. The preferred method presently is to utilize penetrating diathermy as well as cryopexy in the area of the retinal tear or disinsertion. Cryopexy alone may be applied to the remaining quadrants. Sulfur hexafluoride and air are injected into the vitreous cavity to aid in tamponading the retina against the buckle.[6]

RETAINED REACTIVE INTRAOCULAR FOREIGN BODY

The presence of a retained reactive intraocular foreign body may be demonstrated by a combined radiographic and ultrasonic technique.[4] Foreign bodies often produce lens rupture or retinal detachment, and the treatment of these emergencies has already been described; however, clinical demonstration of magnetic properties or the likelihood of a reactive material is an indication for immediate removal of the foreign body.

If the media are opaque (Fig. 12-7) or if the foreign body is incarcerated within a fibroplastic capsule, vitrectomy may be indicated. In these situations the identification of a foreign body and its subsequent removal require sophisticated preoperative planning. In the presence of a magnetic foreign body, I prefer a pars plana incision approximately 90° from the site of the foreign body. By this positioning the route of magnetic extraction is across the vitreous compartment rather than along the surface of the retina, where the foreign body might produce additional retinal or vascular damage. The incision is not made further away than 90° to avoid an overlong distance between the foreign body and the magnet.

In the presence of a nonmagnetic foreign body or a foreign body that has been neglected until fibrosis has bound it to the retina, sufficient clearing of the fibrotic strands attached to the foreign body must be achieved. The introduction of a second instrument into the eye to aid in this peeling of fibrous tissue is often essential. A 22-gauge needle with bent tip, as described by Machemer,[6] allows fibrin to be peeled away from an encapsulated foreign body. The foreign body can then be removed with a magnet or, if nonmagnetic, with the Neubauer forceps under direct visualization in the manner described by Machemer.[6]

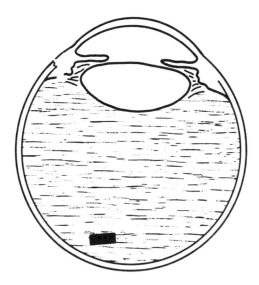

Fig. 12-7. Dense vitreous hemorrhage obscuring a retained reactive intraocular foreign body which requires vitrectomy and removal under direct visualization.

To reinforce the retina against later possible vitreous traction, I generally favor placement of cryopexy over the site of the foreign body. When a full-thickness retinal tear has been found, the use of an explant may also be indicated.

LATE TRAUMA

After perforating injury, dense connective tissue membranes may form in the vitreous, especially along the path of penetration. Often the vitreous compartment is poorly visualized in these cases, not only because of these membranes but also because of the presence of secluded pupil secondary to the original injury. Secondary membranes after cataract extraction also may present as a form of late injury amenable to vitrectomy.

The removal of secondary membranes follows the pars plana procedure as just described. A central opening can be made in the membrane and, since the iris is usually firmly adherent to the membranes, a central iridectomy for visual purposes can also be performed by the vitrectomy instrument. This procedure is usually quite easily performed, with the exception that dense well-organized membranes may not be deformable enough to be aspirated into the cutter opening. In this case special vitreous scissors or blades,[1,2] such as a diamond blade or an ultrasonically vibrated knife, may be useful.

· · ·

Trauma which results in (1) lens rupture, with expulsion of lens material into the vitreous, (2) massive vitreous hemorrhage accompanied by ciliary body laceration or posterior globe perforation, (3) retinal detachment with vitreous hemorrhage, or (4) retained reactive intraocular foreign body often requires vitrectomy. Because of inflammatory vitritis and fibroplastic changes, the earliest possible surgical intervention is recommended in these situations. Removal of lens material, reactive foreign bodies, and traction membranes and early repair of retinal detachment may be facilitated by vitrectomy.

REFERENCES

1. Coleman, D. J.: A diamond knife for vitreous surgery, Trans. Am. Acad. Ophthalmol. Otolaryngol. 76(2):522, 1972.
2. Coleman, D. J., and Everrett, W.: An ultrasonic blade for vitreous surgery. In Irvine, and O'Malley, editors: Proceedings of the Conference on Vitreous Surgery, Springfield, Ill., Charles C Thomas, Publisher. (In press.)
3. Coleman, D. J., and Franzen, L. A.: Vitreous surgery: pre-operative evaluation and prognostic value of ultrasonic display of vitreous hemorrhage, Arch. Ophthalmol. 92:375, 1974.
4. Coleman, D. J., and Trokel, S. L.: A protocol for B-scan and radiographic foreign body localization, Am. J. Ophthalmol. 71(1):84, 1971.
5. Coleman, D. J., Smith, M. E., and Franzen, L. A.: Ultrasonic evaluation of the trans-vitreal trauma. Presented at the nineteenth annual meeting of the American Institute of Ultrasound in Medicine, Seattle, 1974.
6. Machemer, R.: A new concept for vitreous surgery. Part 7, Two-instrument techniques in pars plana vitrectomy, Arch. Ophthalmol. 92:407, 1974.
7. Machemer, R., Buettner, H., and Parel, J-M.: A new concept for vitreous surgery. Part I, Instrumentation, Am. J. Ophthalmol. 73:1, 1972.
8. Parel, J-M., Machemer, R., and Aumayr, W · A new concept for vitreous surgery. Part IV, Improvements in instrumentation and illumination, Am. J. Ophthalmol. 77:6, 1974.

13

Pars plana vitrectomy for conditions other than advanced diabetic retinopathy

EDWARD OKUN

Advanced diabetic retinopathy accounted for ninety of the first 120 vitrectomies performed at Barnes Hospital in 1974 and 1975 (75%). Of the remaining thirty vitrectomies, fifteen were in eyes with traumatic injuries, five in eyes with opacified vitreous hemorrhage secondary to retinal branch vein occlusion, and the remaining ten for a variety of conditions including vitreous hemorrhage secondary to Eales' disease, rhegmatogenous retinal detachment, Kuhnt-Junius macular degeneration, macular detachment secondary to abnormal vitreoretinal traction, and visual loss secondary to residual or displaced lens remnants. The present chapter will attempt to summarize this experience and determine the effectiveness of vitrectomy for these more unusual conditions.

TRAUMA

All but two of the fifteen traumatic cases presented with opacified vitreous hemorrhage. These injuries can be divided into major categories as follows:
1. Perforating injury with sharp object, in and out same wound (knife, wire, jeweler's screwdriver)—3
2. Perforating injury with retained foreign body (gunshot)—1
3. Perforating injury after removal of foreign body—4
4. Double perforating injury—5
5. Contusion injury with ruptured globe after repair—1
6. Contusion injury without ruptured globe—1

Results

Six of the fifteen eyes recovered some useful vision; but only two had 20/70 or better, and in both of these the retinal detachments were repaired—one being a screwdriver injury, the other a double perforating injury. Retinal detachment was a complicating factor in thirteen of the fifteen eyes operated on for trauma. Eight had long-standing retinal detachment uncovered at the time of vitrectomy; and in each instance the detachment was predicted by ultrasound. Two eyes underwent vitrectomy because of known retinal detachment—one a rolled over retina, the other an inferior detachment secondary to traction-induced disinsertion. Three eyes developed postoperative retinal detachment; two of these had suffered double perforating injuries, and one had undergone a successful foreign body extraction prior to opacification of the vitreous. The first two retinas were successfully reattached with scleral buckling procedures. The traction dialysis was successfully closed by first a scleral buckling procedure and then (1 month later) the vitrectomy. It was felt that the disinsertion should be closed first before the fibrovascular ingrowth was severed by vitrectomy, the fear being enlargement and further detachment of the retinal detachment as the infusion fluid worked through the disinsertion. This eye did well, recovering visual acuity of 20/70.

Only one of the eight long-standing retinal detachments uncovered at the time of vitrectomy responded to a combination vitrectomy–scleral buckling procedure. In spite of reattachment, this eye regained only count fingers visual acuity.

Case reports

1. The earliest vitrectomy in this series was performed 3 weeks after a double perforating injury. A large hemorrhage was initially seen immediately temporal and inferior to the macula. Sweet & Comberg x-ray localization had placed the foreign body just outside the sclera. Ultrasound examination confirmed this location. It was hoped that the hemorrhage would clear enough to allow photocoagulation to be applied to the exit site. The vitreous completely opacified over the next 3 weeks. Only a black reflex could be seen, and the injured lens was now turning cataractous.

A combined pars plana lensectomy and vitrectomy cleared the vitreous enough to reveal the tract that the foreign body had made through the vitreous. With minimal effort the fibrous tract was removed. As the retina was approached, there was slight oozing of blood from the amputated end of the tract nearest the exit site. Where it filled the retinal deficit, this stump had the appearance of placental tissue. At the edges the retina appeared smoothly incarcerated into the exit site, so we elected to leave well enough alone. The exit site was approximately one disc diameter temporal to the macula.

On the third postoperative day the retina became detached secondary to leakage through the exit hole. The hole was closed by cryopexy and an episcleral sponge, plus drainage of subretinal fluid (Fig. 13-1, *A*). Three months later the retinal detachment recurred. This time a disinsertion was treated with an encircling procedure. The retina has remained attached. The macula has some striations but visual acuity has returned to 20/100 (Fig. 13-1, *B* and *C*).

2. Three months after a double perforating injury a vitrectomy was performed for the purpose of clearing the vitreous and evaluating the retina, which was shown by ultrasound to be detached. The foreign body tract was easily located. It was very taut and extremely resistant to incarceration into the cutting port. Because of its rubberlike consistency, it could not be severed with the Roto-Extractor. Enough of the vitreous was

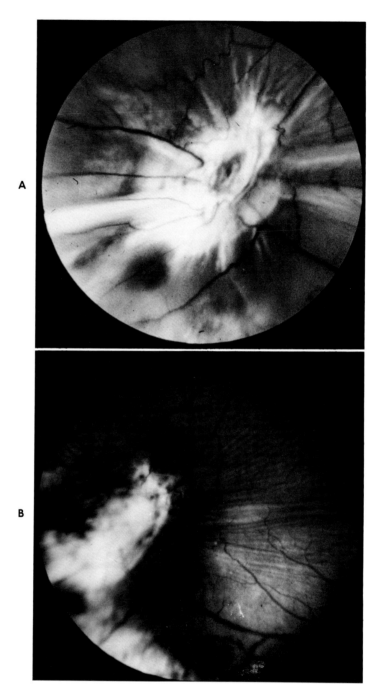

Fig. 13-1. A, Exit site of a foreign body 1 week after a scleral buckling procedure and 2 weeks after a combined lensectomy-vitrectomy for opacified vitreous secondary to a double perforating injury. **B,** Same exit site 9 months after the buckling procedure and 6 months after a second buckling procedure.

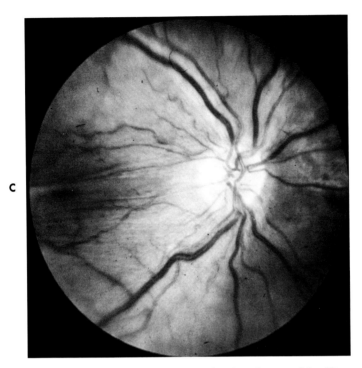

C

Fig. 13-1, cont'd. C, Macula of the same eye 6 months after the second buckling procedure (9 months after the combined lensectomy-vitrectomy).

cleared, however, to uncover the long-standing retinal detachment. Because of the extensive fibrosis and the fixed nature of the retinal detachment, the operation was terminated at this point.

Comment

No two cases of trauma are alike, but experience gained in this series of vitrectomies performed primarily for opacified vitreous hemorrhage secondary to various types of trauma indicates that these hemorrhages should be cleared early. Very few clear spontaneously within a month, and after 2 or 3 months the fibrovascular tracts are too dense to be cut. Retinal detachments associated with perforating trauma are very resistant to therapy once fibrosis has set in—another reason for earlier intervention. Retinal detachments after vitrectomy have a better prognosis than do those uncovered in the course of vitrectomy, probably because fibrosis has not yet set in. Vitrectomy performed earlier than 1 month after an injury can interrupt and eliminate the fibrovascular tracts before they become firmly established and can thus reduce the likelihood of subsequent inoperable traction detachment.

BRANCH VEIN OCCLUSION

Retinal branch vein occlusion was discovered in five eyes after opacified vitreous hemorrhages had been removed. Visual improvement occurred in all five instances. Final visual acuities depended on how badly the macula had been affected. Visual acuities attained in these five eyes were 20/70, 20/80, 20/200, 20/300, and 20/400.

Vitrectomy performed on eyes with opacified vitreous hemorrhage secondary to retinal branch vein occlusion is very similar to that performed for diabetic retinopathy. A similar fibrovascular stalk is usually encountered and the vitreous is similarly cut free from the stalk. These eyes have shown less proliferative involvement than have the eyes of diabetics and they also seem to recover more rapidly. The diagnosis is usually made only after the vitreous hemorrhage has been cleared.

VITREOUS OPACIFICATION SECONDARY TO EALES' DISEASE

Two patients had Eales' disease diagnosed prior to the development of a massive hemorrhage. One eye appeared to have undergone an uncomplicated vitrectomy. On the fourth postoperative day there was a recurrent hemorrhage and the course was downhill from that day on. Not only did the hemorrhage fail to clear, but rubeosis iridis set in. The other patient had an extremely dense organized hemorrhage with multiple membranes seen on preoperative ultrasound examination. Retinal detachment was suspected but the retina was found intact, and 20/400 visual acuity was achieved.

LONG-STANDING VITREOUS HEMORRHAGE SECONDARY TO RHEGMATOGENOUS RETINAL DETACHMENT

Retinal detachments were uncovered in two patients. One was an inoperable fixed detachment of long standing; the other responded to a scleral buckling procedure with visual improvement from hand motion to 20/300.

In certain rare instances, the vitreous hemorrhage suffered at the time of retinal tear formation fails to resorb and thus interferes with definitive therapy of the retinal detachment. If the detachment can be detected by ultrasound or by partial visualization, a very cautious vitrectomy can be undertaken for the purpose of improving visualization to the point at which a scleral buckling procedure can be undertaken.

VITREOUS OPACIFICATION SECONDARY TO K.J. MACULAR DEGENERATION

A subretinal tumor mass was uncovered by this vitrectomy. Malignant melanoma was immediately suspected, and all vitreous cuttings were prepared for histologic study. The retinal elevation was primarily temporal to the fovea and actually split the fovea. The color was yellowish with some areas that appeared speckled brown. Although the retina appeared mottled inferiorly, there was no exudative detachment in this location. Most of the mass was uncovered, care being taken not to cut into it. The cell block prepared from the vitrectomy suction fluid revealed only fibrin and hemoglobin breakdown products. No tumor cells were seen.

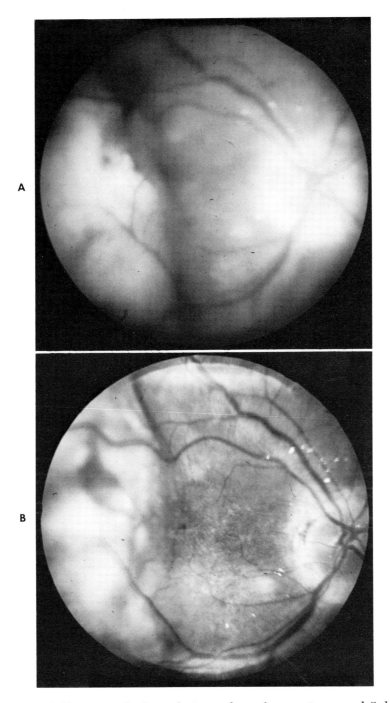

Fig. 13-2. A, Probable organized subretinal vitreous hemorrhage as it appeared 5 days after vitrectomy for opacified vitreous hemorrhage. Malignant melanoma had to be ruled out. **B,** Six months after the vitrectomy. The subretinal mass has shrunken slightly, and visual acuity has improved to count fingers.

On the second postoperative day a ^{32}P test was performed and was negative. Fluorescein angiography was performed on the fifth postoperative day and repeated 6 months postoperatively. Both these angiograms revealed mainly blockage of the underlying choroid. A metastatic x-ray survey and liver scan were negative. Serial fundus photographs have shown shrinkage of the organized subretinal hemorrhage over the past 6 months (Fig. 13-2). Visual acuity has improved from hand motion to count fingers at 2 feet.

In cases of opacified vitreous hemorrhage, one never knows what will be found after the vitreous has been cleared. Ultrasound is of great help, but the definitive answer comes only after the surgery. A tumor should always be suspected; and, if possible, the diagnosis should not be made by cutting directly into it. The ophthalmoscopic appearance, the clinical course, and the additional help gained from ultrasound, ^{32}P, and fluorescein angiography will usually suffice to make the diagnosis. In this instance a valuable eye was saved since the patient's other eye was badly affected by macular degeneration.

VITREOUS TRACTION ON THE MACULA

An abnormally firm ring-shaped vitreoretinal adhesion about the left macula of a 49-year-old woman gradually detached her macula and reduced visual acuity from 20/20 to 20/400 (Fig. 13-3, *A*). The mechanism seemed to be one of a retracting vitreous firmly attached to the macula, and vitrectomy appeared to be the logical treatment. An uncomplicated vitrectomy was performed, and the next day the macula was flat once again. Six months later the visual acuity had returned to 20/30 (Fig. 13-3, *B*).

OPACIFIED LENS REMNANTS OR INFLAMMATION SECONDARY TO DISLOCATED LENS REMNANTS

Four patients were operated on for lens remnants. Two had lens nuclei and cortex dislocated into the vitreous after phacoemulsification procedures, and two had residual membranes (one after trauma, the other after congenital cataract surgery). Each of these lensectomy procedures was associated with a shallow anterior vitrectomy. Since in one patient the dislocated nucleus eventually came to rest on the retina, a fairly complete vitrectomy was performed. The patient recovered 20/60 visual acuity. The uveitis soon came under control, and the intraocular pressure returned to normal. The membranous cataract which had formed secondary to trauma also responded very well; but follow-up has been too short on this patient to be meaningful. The other two patients were known to harbor retinal detachments. The eye with the dislocated nucleus did well with the addition of a scleral buckling procedure. Removal of the congenital membranous cataract revealed a massive preretinal retraction type of detachment that flattened out at first but later recurred.

SUMMARY

1. Trauma accounted for 50% of the nondiabetic eyes' undergoing vitrectomy.

2. Early intervention is advantageous in these cases because of irreversible fibrotic changes that occur between 3 weeks and 3 months after trauma.

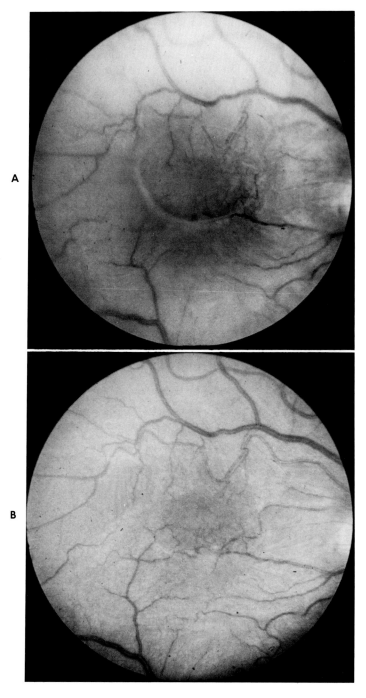

Fig. 13-3. A, Ring-shaped macular detachment secondary to abnormal vitreoretinal adhesion and vitreous retraction. Visual acuity is 20/400. **B,** Six months after vitrectomy. The macula is flat, and visual acuity is 20/30.

3. Underlying the spontaneous vitreous hemorrhage in the nondiabetic eyes were retinal branch vein occlusion (5 eyes), Eales' disease (2 eyes), rhegmatogenous retinal detachment (2 eyes), and K.J. macular degeneration (1 eye). The last is easily confused with malignant melanoma, which may also underlie an organized vitreous hemorrhage.

4. A case of abnormal vitreous traction producing macular detachment was successfully treated by vitrectomy.

5. Pars plana lensectomy-vitrectomy is a satisfactory approach to dislocated lens fragments or residual membranes.

EDITOR'S COMMENT

In the illustrative case of vitreous traction on the macula (Fig. 13-3), it must be kept in mind that this was a most unusual case of persistent dense vitreomacular adhesion with a gradual drop of visual acuity from 20/20 to 20/400 over a 6-month period. Eyes with less dense vitreomacular adhesion may spontaneously improve without surgical intervention. The dramatic result obtained in Dr. Okun's case was rewarding and was achieved with oscillatory cutting by the Roto-Extractor without the use of a second instrument in the eye (i.e., a 22-gauge needle).

14

Complications of vitrectomy

KURT A. GITTER
GERALD COHEN

This chapter is divided into two portions. The first half describes our early experience with microsurgical pars plana vitrectomy in thirty-six consecutive cases performed from July, 1974, to April, 1975, with emphasis on complications incurred. The second half analyzes the recorded complications of 385 consecutive vitrectomies performed by various members of this symposium. A discussion is also included of general and specific techniques to avoid many surgical complications of vitrectomy.

VISUAL RESULTS IN THIRTY-SIX CASES

The visual results and the types of cases treated are shown in Table 14-1. Our best visual results were obtained in anterior chamber reconstruction cases (e.g., cataract, secluded pupil). Diabetic retinopathy with vitreous hemorrhage was the reason why the majority of eyes underwent microsurgical vitrectomy, and visual results in this group were the least favorable. Our complications of vitrectomy in these thirty-six cases included damage to the cornea and lens, retinal tears and detachment, glaucoma, rubeosis, hyphema, vitreous hemorrhage, and intraocular metal shavings. Thirty-four cases were done with the Douvas Roto-Extractor, and two with the Machemer VISC. A list of possible complications of vitrectomy is as follows:

1. Cornea
   a. Corneal edema
   b. Corneal vascularization
2. Lens
   a. Dislocation
   b. Cataract
3. Retina
   a. Retinal tear and/or detachment
   b. Dialysis
4. Glaucoma
5. Hyphema-rubeosis
6. Vitreous hemorrhage
7. Other
   a. Phthisis bulbi
   b. Sympathetic ophthalmia
   c. Iritis
   d. Vitritis
   e. Intraocular retention of metal shavings

Table 14-1. Results of vitrectomy in thirty-six consecutive cases

			Visual acuity	
Preoperative diagnosis	*No.*	*Improved*	*Unchanged*	*Worse*
Postcataract secluded pupil; anterior chamber reconstruction	10	9	1	0
Diabetic retinopathy	16	6	5	5
Branch vein occlusion	4	3	0	1
Trauma	4	2	1	1
Coat's syndrome	1	1	0	0
Pars planitis	1	1	0	0

COMPLICATIONS IN THIRTY-SIX CASES
Cornea

Corneal edema occurred in five cases, and corneal vascularization in one case. The edema persisted in two cases of postoperative rubeosis iridis, both of which ultimately required enucleation for absolute glaucoma. Three other cases of postoperative corneal edema were transient, and in two instances postoperative bullous keratopathy was successfully managed with soft contact lenses.

Lens

Our lens complications included one dislocation, one dispersal of significant amounts of lens material into the vitreous cavity, and one postoperative cataract. A posterior subcapsular cataract developed in one eye of an elderly diabetic patient within a few months after vitrectomy, and it may represent either a complication of the vitrectomy or a routine progression of lens changes in a diabetic eye with early preoperative lens changes.

Retina

Retinal tears and/or detachments occurred in five cases. Iatrogenic tears were created in two diabetic eyes, with traction retinal detachments of the posterior pole when fibrous bands were lysed with the vitrectomy unit. The surgeon must take great care when cutting these fibrotic proliferative bands associated with traction retinal detachments. Cutting the bands directly adjacent to the retina must be avoided since it is easy to produce an iatrogenic tear in this manner.

A retinal tear and detachment also occurred during a combined lensectomy and vitrectomy procedure when, after the lens had become dislocated, the retina inadvertently was torn during attempts to retrieve the dislocated lens. Two other retinal detachments occurred in the postoperative period 1 and 3 months, respectively, after successful vitrectomy procedures. In each eye the postvitrectomy result had been 20/40 or better. A detachment occurred 1 month after a successful vitrectomy in an eye that had suffered a shotgun wound with secondary vitreous hemorrhage. The retina was successfully reattached with an episcleral

no. 40 band and 5 mm sponge over the original scleral laceration. A second patient, referred to us after a successful lensectomy and vitrectomy at the National
Eye Institute for long-standing vitreous hemorrhage, developed a retinal detachment 3 months after the vitrectomy. The visual acuity was correctable to
20/30 after the lensectomy and vitrectomy. The retina was successfully reattached, with preservation of central vision (20/30), after an intrascleral buckling
procedure with diathermy and drainage of subretinal fluid.

It is significant that no retinal dialyses were found in our series of thirty-six
eyes.

IOP elevation

Elevated intraocular pressure occurred in seven cases—five of which were
transient, either inflammatory or hemolytic in nature. Two cases persisted with
rubeosis iridis and absolute glaucoma. Transient postoperative elevations of intraocular pressure were controlled medically with carbonic anhydrase inhibitors
and topical epinephrine.

Hyphema-rubeosis

Postoperative hyphema was present in four eyes but cleared in two cases.
Two were persistent and associated with the postoperative development of

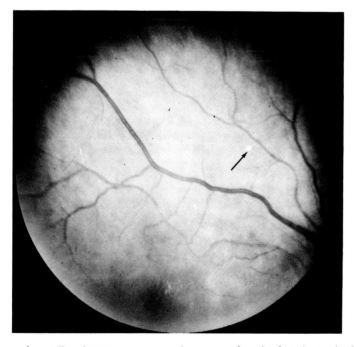

Fig. 14-1. Presumed metallic shaving seen as a glistening refractile disc (arrow) above the
superficial temporal vein.

rubeosis iridis. The postoperative development of neovascular glaucoma may represent further progression of underlying diabetic vascular disease rather than a true complication of vitrectomy. Nevertheless, this development is one of the gravest problems faced in diabetic eyes which undergo vitrectomy.

Other

Other potential complications include phthisis bulbi, sympathetic ophthalmia, and endophthalmitis, none of which occurred in our series. In two diabetic eyes with successful vitrectomy, a glistening refractile presumed metallic shaving, approximately 100 to 200 μm in size, was noted in the posterior pole during the postoperative period (Fig. 14-1). The shaving remained stationary for a year in one eye and for 2 months in the other eye; to date there have been no visible side effects.

ANALYSIS OF COMPLICATIONS IN 385 CASES

To provide a larger selection of patients from which to study rates and types of complication, we requested members of our panel to review their complications of vitrectomy. Accordingly 385 consecutive cases of microsurgical vitrectomy were tabulated from the following authors: Okun—107, Peyman—100, Coleman—60, Federman—55, Gitter and Cohen—36, Kasner—27. The complication parameters that were measured and recorded included glaucoma (transient and persistent), uveitis, recurrent vitreous hemorrhage, corneal changes, retinal tears, detachment and dialysis, rubeosis iridis and phthisis bulbi.

Several categories of ocular disorders were evaluated. These included diabetic vitreous hemorrhages, anterior chamber reconstruction, rhegmatogenous retinal detachment, and traumatic vitreous hemorrhage.

Diabetes

Diabetic eyes were subdivided into those which had vitrectomy (1) with and (2) without lensectomy. The latter group represented either aphakic eyes or phakic eyes with clear lenses. A significantly higher complication rate was found in diabetic eyes that underwent a combined lensectomy-vitrectomy procedure—particularly postoperative rubeosis iridis (17% vs. 6%) and retinal tear, dialysis or detachment (9% vs. 5%) (Tables 14-2 and 14-3). These findings in diabetic eyes suggest that separate surgical procedures for vitrectomy and lensectomy may be preferable.

Complications in our combined lensectomy-vitrectomy cases included retinal tear and detachment, phthisis bulbi, retained lens nucleus, and secondary glaucoma. One of our cases was of particular interest because enucleation was eventually performed and histopathology obtained. Preoperatively this eye had had an organized vitreous hemorrhage present for three years with light perception and projection vision. A combined lensectomy-vitrectomy was performed. It was complicated by partial lens dislocation into the posterior segment. The entire lens nucleus could not be removed, and during the surgery a retinal tear was

Table 14-2. Complications of diabetic pars plana microsurgical vitrectomy with lensectomy (130 cases)

	Percent
Rubeosis iridis	17
Persistent glaucoma	16
Recurrent hemorrhage	13
Retinal tear or detachment	9
Persistent uveitis greater than 2 mo.	9
Corneal breakdown	5
Loss of eye—phthisis	5
Lens particle in vitrectomy	5

Table 14-3. Complications of diabetic pars plana microsurgical vitrectomy without lensectomy (127 cases)

	Percent
Vitreous hemorrhage	10
Glaucoma	9
Postoperative rubeosis	6
Retinal tear or detachment	5
Uveitis	5
Loss of eye	2
Cataracts	2

created. Despite attempts at repair, the eye subsequently developed rubeosis and secondary glaucoma and was enucleated. The histopathology, performed by Dr. Myron Yanoff, at the Scheie Eye Institute, disclosed a thick fibrous membrane adjacent to the ruptured lens capsule which contained blood, pus, and isolated segments of lens cortical material. This was surrounded by a granulomatous reaction containing plasma cells, lymphocytes, epithelioid, and giant cells (phacoanaphylactic reaction) (Fig. 14-2). The eye also had evidence of a retinal detachment and rubeosis iridis.

Anterior chamber reconstruction

Anterior chamber pathology—such as membranous, traumatic, or secondary cataracts, vitreocorneal touch, iris seclusion, and updrawn pupil—have all yielded excellent results with this type of surgery (Table 14-4).

Retinal detachment

Complication rates of vitrectomy in cases of retinal detachment (usually with associated MVR or detachments with severe and long-standing hemorrhage) were high. Recurrent retinal detachment and vitreous hemorrhage occurred in approximately 25% of twenty-six reported cases (Table 14-5). These cases represented last-stage efforts at surgical repair of complicated retinal detachments.

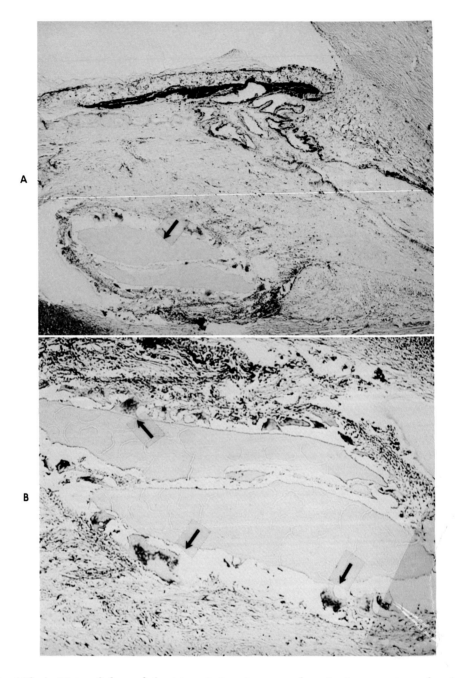

Fig. 14-2. A, Histopathology of the iris, anterior vitreous, and angle demonstrating rubeosis iridis and lens remnants (arrow) in the vitreous surrounded by fibrosis, inflammation, and hemorrhage. **B,** Higher magnification showing giant cells (arrows) surrounding the retained lens remnants.

Table 14-4. Complications of pars plana vitrectomy in secondary or postcataract membranes (58 cases)

	Percent
Transient glaucoma	4
Corneal edema	3
Vitreous hemorrhage	3
Retinal detachment	2

Table 14-5. Complications of microsurgical pars plana vitrectomy in rhegmatogenous retinal detachment (26 cases)

	Percent
Retinal detachment	30
Vitreous hemorrhage	23
Corneal breakdown	8

Table 14-6. Complications of microsurgical pars plana vitrectomy in trauma (43 cases)

	Percent
Recurrent vitreous hemorrhage	16
Retinal detachments	14
Loss of eye—phthisis	12
Persistent glaucoma	7
Persistent uveitis	5

Trauma

The results in trauma cases, depicted in Table 14-6, show a relatively high rate of recurrent vitreous hemorrhage (16%), retinal detachment (14%), and phthisis bulbi (12%)—which is undoubtedly influenced by the severity of the trauma.

Overall

The overall complication rate of the 385 consecutive microsurgical vitrectomies is shown in Table 14-7. Recurrent vitreous hemorrhage, retinal tear and detachment, and the development of postoperative rubeosis iridis were the most frequent complications.

These statistics do not analyze visual results. It is vital to understand that a perfect surgical result from vitrectomy may not affect visual improvement if the underlying integrity of the retina, choroid, vascular supply, and optic nerve is severely compromised. One case of a 12-year-old traumatic cataract in a young adult served as a good example. This eye had good light perception and projec-

Table 14-7. Overall complication rate of 385 microsurgical vitrectomies

	Percent
Recurrent vitreous hemorrhage	13
Retinal tear, dialysis or detachment	12
Postoperative rubeosis iridis	12
Glaucoma greater than 2 mo.	8
Phthisis bulbi or loss of eye	7

tion vision with no fundus view and normal A- and B-scan ultrasound. An uncomplicated pars plana lensectomy-vitrectomy was performed with hopes of an excellent visual result. The postoperative visual acuity, however, could not be improved better than 20/200 due to a preexisting underlying choroidal rupture which traversed the macula and may have been associated with the original trauma.

SUBDIVISION OF COMPLICATIONS
SURGICAL AND NONSURGICAL

Complications of vitrectomy can be subdivided into surgical (those that occur on the operating table) and nonsurgical (those not affected by surgical technique). We, as ophthalmic surgeons, have some control over the former but little if any control over the latter group of complications.

Surgical complications include lens changes—cataract (if not performing a simultaneous lensectomy) and/or dispersal of lens cortical or nuclear fragments (while performing a lensectomy). Other surgically induced complications include corneal endothelial changes, retinal tears, dialysis and detachments, hemorrhage during surgery, and postoperative uveitis and glaucoma.

The nonsurgical considerations are primarily the development of postoperative rubeosis iridis and recurrent vitreous hemorrhage from further neovascularization. These phenomena lead to recurrent hemorrhage and loss of vision and do not appear to be associated with surgical technique.

METHODS OF AVOIDING SURGICAL COMPLICATIONS
General

Proper patient selection and careful preoperative evaluation, as outlined in Chapter 6, are imperative if good visual results and reduced complication rates are to be achieved.

All ophthalmologists interested in performing these procedures must achieve dexterity using a binocular operating microscope with coaxial illumination and zoom control. Because of the frequent association of tears, detachments, and/or dialysis in many of these eyes, the vitreous surgeon should also be capable of performing retinal detachment surgery.

Vitreous surgeons should be knowledgeable in all aspects of posterior segment disorders and should have a thorough understanding of fluorescein angiography, electrophysiology, and ultrasonography.

The neophyte vitreous surgeon should be aware, furthermore, that his initial cases will yield significantly higher complication rates—which will decrease as familiarity with technique and skills is developed.

Specific

Certain specific surgical techniques can be employed and learned to reduce the hazards of complications:

1. *Control of intraocular bleeding during and after surgery.* During vitrectomy the surgeon can usually control intraocular bleeding by regulating intraocular pressure. He does this by raising and lowering the Ringer's solution bottle and controlling the input and output of fluids. Large-diameter vessel stalks which continue to bleed may require intraocular cauterization via diathermy. After vitrectomy, photocoagulation of persistent new vessels will sometimes prevent further vitreous hemorrhage.

2. *Method of entry and removal of the vitrectomy unit.* It is mandatory that a snug fit be achieved to ensure adequate suction during vitrectomy and to maintain proper control of intraocular pressure during and at the completion of the procedure.

   After entering the midvitreous cavity using a stab incision with an appropriately sized Graefe knife (Machemer type), we preplace a mattress suture at the scleral entry site. We then introduce the vitrectomy instrument with its fiber-optic attachment into the vitreous cavity, using fixation forceps on the anterior scleral lip. The instrument remains in the eye until the termination of the vitrectomy.

   To attain good suction capability for aspiration and easy control of intraocular pressure by fluid regulation, our entry wound is made to fit tightly. On removal of the instrument, the mattress sutures are tied securely—thereby avoiding hypotony and intraocular hemorrhage.

This method of single entry may also account for a reduced incidence of retinal dialysis. Some manufacturers of equipment have developed trochars and cannulas to achieve the effect of a single entry procedure.

3. *Separation of lensectomy and vitrectomy.* In our opinion this seems to be justified. The length of the procedure is significantly reduced, and postoperative complications lessened. Although our statistics substantiate this idea, other men, including Machemer, have strongly advocated using a combined lensectomy-vitrectomy procedure.

The nonsurgical complications of recurrent neovascularization (particularly in diabetic retinopathy) and the development of rubeosis are difficult problems. Perhaps early vitrectomy will prove useful in eyes with proliferative diabetic retinopathy. This question may be answered in the forthcoming N.I.H. clinical trial of early vitrectomy.

Eyes with proliferative retinopathies may significantly benefit by photocoagulation after successful vitrectomy.

The development and cause of rubeosis iridis are a subject of continued importance and interest. It may be that many eyes with preexisting rubeosis iridis were undetected until after surgery. Further analysis of the causes of development of rubeosis, particularly in diabetics, is required.

Round table discussion
Chapters 8 to 14

Peyman We'll start with simple questions that sometimes arise. I would like the panel to respond to this question. How long would you wait to perform vitrectomy in a diabetic patient suffering from vitreous hemorrhage? That means how soon would you perform vitrectomy?

Okun I think it depends on the total situation. If they have one eye functioning well, then I'd give at least a year for the hemorrhage to clear. This is in an eye where you can't see anything. If an ultrasound examination reveals a retinal detachment or the symptomatology indicates not just a retinal break but a retinal detachment also, then I think I would go in earlier, probably at the time I made that diagnosis by ultrasound to see whether or not I could help that situation along. If both eyes are blind, then it's my policy to go in at about 6 months.

Peyman In your experience, Dr. Okun, does vitreous hemorrhage which hasn't cleared in 6 months clear by waiting another 6 months?

Okun I've seen vitreous hemorrhages clear at 6 months, one year, two years, three years, and five years with pretty good visual function thereafter. Unfortunately, I can't predict which will; but I've certainly had in the office prior to the days of vitrectomy some of my early photocoagulation patients who had a blind eye on one side. Years later, the blind eye became the better eye after clearance of the vitreous hemorrhage. It's taken perhaps as long as five years to clear.

Douvas I agree with that last statement. I operated on a patient two years ago and was getting ready to do his second eye; it was a similar situation, and, by gosh, he cleared without me. That was two years later—so there is late clearing, but you can't predict these cases. Otherwise, I wait one year for the process to run out. However, many times the history is inaccurate and the patients aren't sure whether or not they have had recurrent hemorrhages. If I see bright blood, I'm more apt to wait for additional clearing. If it all looks yellow, then perhaps there haven't been recurrent intermittent hemorrhages.

Peyman   The next question is directed to Dr. Okun—Would you advise a prophylactic vitrectomy in a diabetic patient with 20/25 vision with or without a
preretinal membrane? Please explain.

Okun   In a diabetic without any preretinal membrane and a visual acuity of
20/25, I'd look the rest of the eye over and see whether I thought it was a
candidate for photocoagulation; but vitrectomy would be the last thing on
my mind. The 20/25 type eye that I showed with massive ingrowth of proliferative tissue or a 20/25 type eye with a proliferative fibrovascular membrane which is undergoing repeated vitreous hemorrhages and having occasional interval vision of 20/25, but fogging to count fingers every so often,
is a different type of eye. I think this type of patient is still somewhat in the
air and I want to stress that it's entirely investigational at this stage as to
whether or not vitrectomy should be performed. I'm very cautiously performing vitrectomy in some of these patients.

My warning is that recurrent vitreous hemorrhage has been a common
complication in these patients with active angiopathy and I think we have to
very carefully evaluate the effectiveness of underwater diathermy in trying
to reduce the angiopathic element. With that, it might be possible to do
earlier vitrectomy and it may be the thing to do. This may, at one time in the
future, become the single most frequent indication for which vitrectomy is
performed. But certainly not today, not yet.

Peyman   Is it your impression that intravitreal stalks regress after vitrectomy?

Okun   I've had the opportunity to reenter two eyes, and neither of these eyes
had had underwater diathermy and both were quite vascular; and when I
reentered them, they were much less vascular and the stalks seemed to regress. I think there is an increased rate of fibrosis and retraction following
vitrectomy; that is, you can leave a stalk perhaps 2 mm long and watch it
gradually retract and become 1 mm after a year to a year and a half.

Peyman   This question is directed to Dr. Gitter. What would be your advice
to a practitioner starting vitrectomy?

Gitter   I'd let Dr. Douvas answer that. He has had so much more experience
than I.

Douvas   Well, obviously, when you look over complication rates, you see the
complications are less in the anterior segment cases, so I would say get the
feel of your instrument if possible, by handling a soft fluffy traumatic cataract.
The next thing would be to start on an aphakic eye with vitreous hemorrhage, preferably an old yellowish one—nothing with bright red blood in it—
and feel your way along that way until you feel comfortable and secure. Go
into lensectomy on the adult cases at a later stage, when you're more secure
with what you're doing.

Gitter   I'd like to comment in one regard. After taking Nick's course in Port
Huron and coming home with the machine and doing several dozen rabbits
and several monkeys and thinking I had the procedure down at least mechanically, and knowing how to use an operating microscope, all I can say is that

it's a lot different in the human eye and it is like every other procedure that everyone has to learn. I think there'll be mistakes when you start doing it, just as when a resident starts doing cataract surgery. Ultimately, I believe the qualifications of a vitreal surgeon include almost all aspects of ophthalmology —namely surgical dexterity, ability to master the operating microscope, and significant knowledge and capability in disorders of the posterior segment including retinal detachment surgery, flourescein angiography, and diagnostic ultrasonography.

Ryan   I think, just to emphasize what Kurt said in his presentation, namely, that you have to be aware of the high complication rate, we had a 30% retinal complication rate, of which about two thirds were retinal dialyses. To me the key to that is that you recognize, first, you have your high index of suspicion. Secondly, at the close of each procedure you do scleral depression of that eye and examine the ora for 360° and obviously be prepared to fix the dialysis or whatever retinal problem you might find at that time. The key factor is that after we demonstrated the high incidence of retinal complications there were only four cases that led to disaster as far as the eye was concerned; so obviously we fixed the majority of them. I don't think we can overemphasize that.

Coleman   I agree very much with Dr. Douvas in terms of the procedure to follow. I'd like to raise the question again on the complication rate that the overall statistic showed. Machemer's reports have shown that in the combined lensectomy with vitrectomy in diabetics there're less complications with the removal of the lens (and this is a much larger group than even Dr. Gitter's combined group of 370 cases) so that, routinely, he advocated removal of the lens in diabetics. I feel that, with exceptions, when there are some with a very clear lens and certainly you feel you can leave the lens, lensectomy and vitrectomy should be simultaneous. One other feature that should be mentioned is rubeosis.

Recently at the meeting in Vail, Colorado, the question of rubeosis has been a major complication, and this might be related to the lens part of the procedure. If we remove the lens, many of these patients develop rubeosis before coming back for the vitrectomy; so it's certainly something to keep in mind that this may be related to the problem. I think lensectomy is going to be required in most of these patients.

Gitter   That's why I really wanted this panel to discuss the complication rates that were found. What I meant by those statistics was lensectomy and vitrectomy combined at one sitting yielded a higher incidence of complications than when separated. I think most lenses have to be removed also. In our very limited experience, we seem to favor the idea of having the lens removed first and then following with a vitrectomy 1 or 2 months later. In fact, some vitreous hemorrhages show remarkable clearance after the lens is removed. There's a higher complication rate of secondary glaucoma, rubeosis, uveitis, etc., if done simultaneously. I'd like to know what the others say.

Okun   I think that we have to think of the condition that we are treating and, of course, diabetes and diabetic hemorrhages are the number one thing. When I reviewed the lensectomies performed for diabetic hemorrhages, we found that we were performing a lensectomy in thirty-six out of forty patients who had lenses at the time of vitrectomy; that is, thirty-six out of forty that had lenses with a diagnosis of organized vitreous hemorrhage had a lensectomy performed at the same time. The reason for this is that there already was some cataract present, perhaps not enough to warrant a cataract extraction by ordinary criteria, but usually at least posterior subcapsular changes, and we felt we were doing a much better vitrectomy with the lens out. There were four people in whom we did not remove the lens. Three of those had recurrent vitreous hemorrhages. Recurrent vitreous hemorrhage in this group has certainly not been a problem.

It has absolutely amazed me that how few of the patients who had a combination lensectomy-vitrectomy for organized hemorrhage have had recurrent vitreous hemorrhage. Now, that is one thing. The next point is that when you take your diabetics who have traction retinal detachment or the diabetics who have retinitis proliferans they have clear lenses. I've not been taking those lenses out because they haven't had the hemorrhage, and the hemorrhage must be important in that pathogenesis of posterior subcapsular change. In those I've noted a recurrent vitreous hemorrhage with the lenses left in place. Nevertheless, we feel that with underwater diathermy we might be able to avoid that. With regard to the complications of rubeosis, it was brought home to me when on 2 successive weeks I had patients scheduled for vitrectomy whom I had sent out for lens extraction previously and they both came back with advanced rubeosis which I didn't recognize prior to their having their lens extraction. It occurred to me that perhaps it isn't our vitrectomy that's causing the rubeosis. Probably it's the trauma to the eye of removing the lens or opening up the vitreous to the anterior chamber or something else other than the straight vitrectomy.

When I broke down straight cases of rubeosis that we had, I was really flabbergasted that only one of eighteen patients who were previously aphakic prior to vitrectomy developed new rubeosis as compared to eight of thirty-three who had a combined lensectomy-vitrectomy. That told me that probably certain patients are at risk at the time they have their lens removed. If we want to find out what that group is, perhaps what we should do is what Kurt has deduced from these studies. Perhaps the lens should be removed earlier and let them percolate for 3 months to see if that is the type of eye that's going to develop rubeosis; and then, if it is, we have to decide if there's too much rubeosis to go ahead—if it's florid rubeosis or if we can treat it. Perhaps do a cyclocryopexy or treat it in some way and proceed with the vitrectomy if you feel it's absolutely essential.

Peyman   What is the incidence of post-op corneal edema, how can it be prevented, and how can it be treated after vitrectomy?

Ryan I think I can speak since we started off with a tremendous incidence of corneal complications. By that, I mean in the first group of patients 60% had transient corneal edema and problems. Overall, I can't remember exactly; this statistic has been reduced to 5% or 10% that have persistent corneal problems. Probably the major factor that we were able to eliminate was the operative or surgical phase of this—namely, by decreasing operating time and decreasing local mechanical trauma to the corneal endothelium.

The way to decrease the trauma is to remove the lens "within the bag" and leave the anterior capsule as long as one can. This takes the extreme with Ron Michels, who will leave this to the very end of the operation, whereas others take out the anterior capsule at the removal of the rest of the lens. I personally leave the anterior capsule until it becomes a factor in visualization of the vitreous and/or retina. In other words, as long as I'm able to operate comfortably, I'll leave that anterior capsule and then remove it subsequently.

Hank Edlehauser has done some exquisite laboratory work in devising the best fluid for irrigation and has determined substances such as glutathione-reinforced Krebs-Ringer's lactate solution seems to be the best. This is going to be commercially available from Alcon. Again this is a factor, but the major thing that we've been able to eliminate (and we don't have these problems any longer) is the operative trauma on a straight mechanical basis.

I should've pointed out that there are two very different populations, the diabetic versus the nondiabetic, with regard to corneal problems. In diabetic patients there is poor adherence of the corneal epithelium to the basement membrane so that after removing that epithelium (if you have to scrape the epithelium) they are going to have much more in the way of problems of recurrent corneal erosion than are the nondiabetics.

Peyman In my experience there has been a direct relationship with the length of procedure and the development of corneal edema. Is that also your experience?

Ryan Yes, with these other factors understood.

Coleman I agree with all that. One other minor thing in avoiding the epithelial scraping, I think that the smaller contact lens is a big clue. The earlier use of the Goldmann lens, which is very large, I think, required more scraping of the cornea. We've used a very small Cardona lens. I understand Duncan and Walk are making a small one also. It's only 8 mm across and there's better perfusion of the anterior cornea; and we don't need to scrape the epithelium ready at all.

Okun One other factor in corneal edema is the frequent relation to increased pressure within the eye. This should be checked. Many times, if you do find the pressure elevated, treat it and the edema will clear. I've had patients where I checked the pressure, found it normal, and then I assumed that that was not the factor in the recurrent erosins and chronic edema; and then a little later on, I rechecked the pressure and found it elevated. When I lowered the pressure by medical management, then every thing took care of itself.

Peyman   In patients who have post-up corneal edema, I use glucose or sodium chloride.

Gitter   We've used therapeutic soft lenses in about four or five cases with post-op corneal edema, with very good results.

Peyman   Dr. Ryan, you describe four cases of endophthalmitis. What organisms were cultured in these four cases?

Ryan   In point of fact, we didn't culture the organism in any of them. We did demonstrate the organism to be a staph type by smear. All of these patients had been previously placed on intravenous antibiotics so I don't think it's surprising that we haven't cultured the organism; but as I say, we have demonstrated the organism by smear.

Peyman   This question is to the panel—Are metallic particles found intraocularly postvitrectomy? How often? What instruments are used?

Douvas   I'll start. On our instrument, occasionally you'll see what I call molecular-size crystals. They are pinpoint things, not shavings, that look like a glistening cholesterol crystal and I'm sure they're particles coming from the instrument. We also did tests by putting Millipore filters on the back of the instrument and pulled considerable fluid through the instrument and did collect some fine pinpoint particles on the filter. Then we did similar tests with plain disposable needles and picked up a few particles that way. The particles are stainless steel, inert, and cause no problem to date. I have yet to see a true shaving, but the molecular crystals I've occasionally noted.

Peyman   From my experience, I have not had particles (that were visible) with my instrument. Any other comments?

Peyman   Question to the panel. What solution do you use for vitrectomy; sodium chloride, Ringer's, lactate Ringer's?

Coleman   I use lactated Ringer's.

Ryan   We are in the process of a controlled series where every other patient is getting a Ringer's solution and the others are getting the glutathione Krebs-Ringer solution, and it wouldn't really be fair to say anything yet except I am convinced that the lighter solution really is causing a little bit less in terms of increasing corneal thickness postoperatively. We are making post-op corneal thickness measurements in all of these patients.

Douvas   I do not have that available and I'm using nonlactated Ringer's, as is Bob Machemer.

Peyman   I personally use sodium chloride and 5% dextrose. Is that the same as you Kurt?

Gitter   We use Ringer's.

Peyman   When the lens nucleus becomes luxated post-phacoemulsification or -lensectomy, should the nucleus always be removed? How so?

Gitter   One of the reasons I personally thought it might be better to do cataracts by standard techniques (separated from the vitrectomy) and then come to the vitrectomy is because we had a high incidence of complications doing combined lensectomy and vitrectomy at the outset. Either the whole nucleus or a good portion of it can be dislocated to the back of the eye. Gerald Cohen showed you one case that originally was a salvageable eye. It was a vein occlusion with three years of hemorrhage, and I'm sure it could have been a good result rather than a tragic one. In that instance the nucleus fell back and I tried to get it with the Roto-Extractor. I then came in from the opposite side with a 22-gauge needle and somehow produced a retinal tear and detachment and could not remove the entire dislocated lens nucleus. On other occasions, I've left some very small portions of nuclear material in the posterior segment without any complications that I've been aware of.

Okun Wasn't your question related to post-phacoemulsification or postextracapsular extraction? The thing that falls back with that procedure, I think, potentially is very dangerous material. I think it's not like a cleaned-off hard part of the nucleus but as cortical material or as nucleus with a lot of cortical material, and I've seen three of these now and they really have very hot eyes. There's a lot of inflammation and glaucoma, and I think that, yes, you should go back and get those out as soon as it seems feasible to go back in on these eyes. I would try and quiet them down as best you can with steroids, then just as soon as I could, go back in, probably within a week or so. If it's a phaco, you certainly could go in very fast.

Coleman I agree completely with Ed following phaco. I've had, I think, a total of three eyes that have lost lens material in the back following phaco. Two of these were just routine phacoemulsification. One was the very first one I did. This was a hot eye with glaucoma, and I agree that this is not just nuclear material. It's usually some cortical material, and these are very bad. In that eye I went back in and irrigated everything out, and the eye turned out 20/20 vision with no real problem. Actually all three eyes came out well, but they were quite inflamed. I think that with this combined procedure, however, using the phaco and the Roto-Extractor through the pars plana, it's not usually a difficult problem if you lose some lens material. I do feel that it's the very dense nucleus where you get the problem, when the phako starts battering the lens nucleus around. It's on the basis of these other cases that I use the needle through the other pars plana, impaling the nucleus to hold it, and that avoids this problem. I haven't had a problem with any breaking of the posterior capsule scaffold (that I like to keep intact when I've impaled it).

Douvas As far as the extracapsular cases, where, say, an attempted intracapsular results with a full section, those I possibly stall for 6 to 8 weeks, depending on the operative reaction and whether there's phacolytic glaucoma that forces your hand. I think this may also be a factor in your phacoemulsification. Of course, you have a smaller incision so you can go in earlier in those cases. There again, I think it's a case of whether they're getting so much operative reaction that you want to intervene early. As far as the routine lensectomy, with the Roto-Extractor technique, occasionally yes, I will luxate particles, but usually if I haven't misjudged the lens in its degree of nuclear sclerosis, that really is no problem removing it from the posterior area. It's usually softened enough that we can aspirate it into the instrument and cut it without having to intervene with the second instrument. However, I have misjudged on two occasions and have had to go in with the second instrument, without complications. I have yet to leave a nucleus of any significance within the eye. Bob Machemer has left, in his early experience, nuclei within the eye devoid of cortex and an eye essentially devoid of vitreous with no operative complication from this. So apparently, it doesn't have to be removed under those circumstances.

Ryan Just to second what everyone has said, I remember well as a resident hearing Dr. Maumenee comment that in his experience at Wilmer he had never seen a case survive where the nucleus had been dropped back into the vitreous cavity. Again, not saying that any of us want to see a large number of such cases, but the point is that whatever it is about that nucleus and the amount of cortex that is wrapped around it, certainly in combination with vitreous it leads to a tremendous inflammation. Then the point that you all have made here, as far as what we encounter at operation with vitrectomy, we can remove the nucleus; and I personally also have not had to leave significant nuclear material in. As has been pointed out, those three cases that Bob Machemer initially reported, those eyes all did well.

Gitter In our complication talk we did show that one slide that Myron Yanoff, of the University of Pennsylvania, read as a phacoanaphylactic reaction surrounding retained lens nucleus in the midvitreous cavity.

Peyman What is the cause of postvitrectomy glaucoma, and how does one treat it?

Okun It's a matter of conjecture as to what you think is causing it. It is there and we see it fairly often. It could be just the prostaglandins that are released with trauma. We have alternatively treated a series of eyes with aspirin to see if we could intercede in that traumatic aspect of the glaucoma.

Hemolytic glaucoma is another mechanism, and we've seen eyes where hemoglobin breakdown products and hemoglobin clogged the trabeculae. Certainly, if an adequate lensectomy is not done and if lens material is left in the eye, we all know that postextracapsular lens extraction or hypermature lenses can plug an angle pretty well. We follow the tensions of patients daily. That may not be great for the epithelium, but we use a Shiøtz tonometer, and it seems to not interfere with corneal healing.

We must also never forget about rubeosis. In eyes that develop rubeosis, it's very interesting that some will have a tremendous rise in intraocular pressure before the rubeosis is clinically appreciated and then the rubeosis shows up later. I'm sure there must be other mechanisms as well. In terms of what you can do for it, I think it should always be treated. I think the corneas, particularly in diabetics, are sick enough that we don't want to allow elevated intraocular pressure to make them still sicker, particularly the endothelium. Diabetics do not tolerate Diamox very well, and you must be extremely careful with these patients because frequently they are on some antihypertensive medication which also can cause potassium loss. I've had several patients almost die when they have gone back to maybe slightly less competent internists and find that they are vomiting because of the Diamox. They're losing potassium and their diabetes gets completely out of control. Anything that can be done to decrease the 2-or-3-week post-op period when there is ocular hypertension would be very much appreciated; and I think anything that can be tried is worthwhile. We use Epinephrine as the drop of choice along with the Diamox; and if Diamox is not tolerated, we employ Naptazane.

Douvas Glaucoma has not been a real problem for me postoperatively. I've had a few and the ones that have been a problem to me are those that are associated with rubeosis and rebleed. Perhaps it hasn't been a significant problem for me because I do a fairly extensive prophylactic cryotherapy to the sclerotomy area using a double-row arc behind it; and maybe, in essence, I'm producing mild cyclocryotherapy along with my routine.

Kasner What are the post-op visual results in PHPV? I can tell you from three cases that the eyes look beautiful but they don't see. The retinas look beautiful and they don't see. Has anybody else found anything different?

Ryan I think that's the essence of it. In six cases that Ron Smith reviewed, one achieved a visual acuity of 20/200. I think our argument for operating is to prevent collapse of the anterior chamber and glaucoma. One of the fellows with Marshall Parks recently told me that he had just operated on an individual in the first 6 months of life with PHPV and claims a 20/40 visual result now. I cannot believe that.

Kasner Dr. Okun, does vitrectomy have any place in massive vitreous retraction therapy?

Okun I wish I could answer that question. I've tried vitrectomy in some cases, but I must admit that I haven't as yet used the two-needle technique or the two-instrument technique. I just don't know. Bob Machemer has, as you know, great courage and has operated on something like thirty patients with MVR, all doing poorly, and with not a single success until he finally got one that succeeded; and now he has stated that his last five were successful. It may be that he's really getting pretty good at picking those membranes off in the earlier stages. I would have to answer, not from my own experience but from what Dr. Machemer says, probably yes.

When I reviewed my own retinal detachment data, I found many patients with early MVR. I'd venture a guess that at least 50% of them are successfully reattached with a buckling procedure, sometimes requiring an intravitreal push. I think what remains to be done is a really good study comparing scleral buckling procedures with these intravitreal procedures for early MVR.

With well-established MVR, I haven't been successful with vitrectomy. I've managed to flatten a few with a combination of vitrectomy and buckling and gas injections. Postoperatively they have come back up again and I wish I had something somewhat less toxic than silicone oil, but something like it, that would be permanent to hold the retina in place. Perhaps vitrectomy will have some role in removing the silicone oil after it has done its job. I haven't been successful in removing it completely. I notice that Dr. Peyman has done one case of vitrectomy and silicone removal, and perhaps we'll see more of this type of treatment for MVR.

Kasner Just for a change of pace, which surgical method is considered best for vitreal touch—a limbal approach with the Roto-Extractor to clear the anterior chamber of vitreous or a pars plana approach with a posterior vitrectomy?

Ryan I think Dr. Douvas and I went by this yesterday—that I'd rather go through the pars plana and I think Dr. Douvas would rather go through the limbus. It would probably be 50-50.

Douvas Primarily, I'm an anterior segment surgeon who does retinas, and I think Dr. Ryan is primarily a retinal surgeon who does anterior segments. My feeling is that the limbal incision, where your instrument is always in your view, is safer, assuming you have a healthy cornea. If you don't have a healthy cornea where you enter the globe, I too would go through the pars plana.

Kasner Where can SF_6 gas be gotten? I think the answer to that is you can't get it because it's not FDA approved and you have to have some kind of permission to use it in this country. But you can go to Canada and bring a case back. Is that the way it works?

Douvas Has the use of air been FDA approved?

Ryan Anyone can apply for an FDA investigational right to use the SF_6 and anyone can purchase SF_6 without any of this. It is used, as most of you know, for making electrical switches and that type of thing. The real question is your own jeopardy of using it without FDA approval. There are several sources of supply in this country, including Allied Chemical, in New Jersey, and Air Products, in Pennsylvania.

Kasner By show of hands, has anyone eaten up a whole retina? (Two panelists.) Has anyone eaten up half a retina? A quarter retina? (Six panelists.) What's the approximate incidence of retinal dialysis?

Coleman The only cases of retinal dialysis I've had have been in trauma (two cases).

Okun Assuming that the eyes that have detachments and you can't find the break are dialysis hidden by the vitreous base, I'd say somewhere in the vicinity of 8% to 10% of cases.

Ryan We ran a 17% evidence of retinal dialysis, and I think this is in part related to how tight we made our incision. I know that, as I'm trying to listen to what Dr. Coleman said about not being impressed with the need for hav-

ing a very tight fit around where you insert the instrument, when one considers the difference in incidence of dialysis it's a rational approach.

Douvas About 8% dialysis.

Gitter We're unaware of any retinal dialysis in our patients, but we are certainly going to look a little harder. This brings up another subject: How
wide a vitrectomy do you perform and how wide must the clear tunnel
created by vitrectomy be? It's very difficult for us to get all the way out and
visualize the anterior retina after we've done a vitrectomy, as our major
concern is only to provide a clear tunnel for vision and not remove all the
organized material within the vitreous cavity. Perhaps by not using the
Roto-Extractor at the area of the vitreous base we've inadvertently not produced retinal dialysis.

Peyman I'd like to mention that in 170 vitrectomy cases, I haven't had a single
dialysis. This may be due to many factors. I've never made a tight wound.
The first 100 vitrectomies were done without a fiber-optic. I didn't push the
fiber-optic inside the eye. It might be somewhat related to the cutting action of
the instrument, which in my instrument has a linear oscillation.

Okun I think dialysis is a terribly important subject and at least in my hands
is a real complication. I think it has an awful lot to do with how well you
place your instrument in the eye. I think one of the really weak points in the
design of the instrument is the right angle shoulder of the light pipe. If you're
not extremely careful with how you get that instrument into the eye, you're
probably going to do things that can lead to dialysis (i.e., pushing the
choroid and vitreous ahead of the instrument, thereby increasing vitreous
traction).

One of the things I've noticed is fewer dialyses in our last fifty cases than
in our first fifty. I think we should really look at our surgical opening to be
sure it is absolutely clear and clean all the way in with an adequate opening
to introduce the vitrectomy unit. Nevertheless, I want it to be extremely
tight because I feel I have an uncontrolled vitrectomy when there's leakage
of fluid coming out of my vitrectomy site. This is particularly important
when it comes to closing leaking blood vessels during vitrectomy.

The other thing besides getting the instrument cleanly into the eye is
freeing up the vitreous from your light pipe once you enter the globe. There
are two maneuvers, both of which Nick taught me: One is to turn the instrument about 360 degrees and continue cutting through the vitreous base.
Never push your instrument all the way across if you've got vitreous fibrils
caught in it because obviously those fibrils are connected to the pars plana
and retina on the opposite side. The other thing is to stay away from the
vitreous base. You really don't have to get too close to the vitreous base for
anything.

I can tell you about dialyses that have occurred on the table. They've usually occurred when I'm around the vitreous base. I think the instrument is cutting well in a rotating cycle, and maybe it's not cutting so well at that time, and

possibly something is getting pulled in at that time. Certainly an instrument that's not cutting very well can be another reason for dialysis along with a poor entry. I think that working without the light pipe will also lower the incidence of dialysis.

Gitter   What about the multiple entries, in and out? Don't you think that has an effect.

Okun   Absolutely, I agree with Kurt 100%. Once I'm in the eye, I will not come out until I finish the operation.

Douvas   The main thing I wanted to bring up was the question of the use of a trocar. We apparently both leave a larger opening. I don't really feel uncomfortable with a wound that's larger. I make a large opening in the vitreous and I think it reduces the complications. I'm going to go for the use of the trocar which Bob Machemer described. I think expanding the wound with the trocar can avoid many of these problems.

Coleman   I agree. I think we should give greater attention to the technique of our sclerotomy. You can make a knife incision; but if you don't follow the precise path of the knife incision with your vitrectomy instrument, then you're still making a blunt pass and having that dilated with a trocar. I think it's going to be very helpful. If you're doing a combined lensectomy-vitrectomy after removing your capsule, you might go ahead and do a fairly shallow anterior vitrectomy at that point as you don't need your light pipe for this maneuver. After clearing some of this area anteriorly, the introduction of the vitrectomy unit and light pipe is made easier.

As Dr. Okun mentioned on the use of 360-degree rotation to cut vitreal fibers, I actually pull the cutting tip inside the light pipe and cut within the light pipe, rotating inside almost 360 degrees in order to cut the fibrous loops internally. So I'm pulling the instrument in and out of the light pipe while I'm rotating until I can see the tissue drop away from the light pipe before I proceed deeper into the eye. Otherwise, if there's vitreous incarcerated between the probe tip and the light pipe and you shove ahead, all you're doing is ripping off the vitreous base, thereby producing a detachment.

Kasner   What's the incidence of patients with rubeosis who have previously had laser therapy? Is there any increased or decreased incidence of rubeosis in eyes that have had laser surgery?

Okun   It has been the experience of some people that after doing pan-retinal ablative treatment, particularly in the periphery with photocoagulation, rubeosis can disappear. I had that happen with one patient who had a central retinal vein occlusion and 100 days later developed rubeosis. I photocoagulated all the way around and had the patient come back 3 weeks later and was absolutely amazed that the rubeosis had disappeared. I can remember my chart because there was a great big "Amazing" on it. I shipped the patient around to be seen and wrote a letter to referring physicians saying how bright I was that I knew about this latest thing. The problem was that the patient came back 2 months later with the rubeosis returned just about as bad as it was initially.

Kasner   Dr. Peyman, you said your machine is disposable. Please explain and tell us what is the advantage of this.

Peyman   The whole instrument, the tip and the one that you hold in your hands and the tubes, everything is disposable. The advantages of having a disposable instrument are numerous. First of all, you always have a backup, and you don't need a full instrument to do another vitrectomy. You always have something available if you need to do a second case or, for that matter, any number of cases that you wish to do. You don't spend time cleaning instruments before and after an operation, and you don't have to worry about sterility in that regard.

Kasner   Dr. Douvas, what camera, film, and light source do you use for your external photographs? What's the secret to your beautiful shots?

Douvas   Get in competition with Bob Machemer. Bob and I play one-upmanship, and he's one-upped me all the way lately. We are closing in. The secret is this—no. 1, use a 30/70% beam splitter so 70% of the light goes to the camera and 30% goes to the surgeon. My light source happens to be the Zeiss Fiber-Optic Light Box. There are going to be even brighter ones available. The question is, do they really increase the output at the light pipe; and Ed Okun tells me it does. The rest of it is optics.

Kasner   Excuse me. When 30% of the light is coming to you, to the surgeon, do you like working in the dark like that?

Douvas   I'm not in the dark. The resolution for me in the human eye is so much greater than the camera. I work along this way all the time so I'm not used to anything more. I can see all right.

   We use high-speed Ektachrome film ASA 125 Tungsten. There are three photoadapters available for the Zeiss scope; one is a 137 photoadapter, a 107, and a 74. The 74 supposedly is to be used for Super-8, but we use if for 16 mm. Your wide open "S" stop on a 137 is an F8. On the 107 it's an F7, and on the 74 it's an F4. So the difference between a 137 and a 74 is two F stops. Two F stops means this: there is a doubling for one F stop and another doubling for the second F stop. You've got a geometric fourfold difference in exposure there. So that means, if you want the greatest advantage of exposure, then you go to a 74 mm adapter.

   The next thing is your working distance or your objective on your microscope. You can work with a 150 mm objective, a 175, or a 200. There's a difference of one F stop between each one of those objectives. You lose two F stops in illumination if you go to a 200 mm objective as opposed to 150. The disadvantage of 150 is you've only got a 6-inch clearance between the botton of the microscope and the eyeball. You are more apt to hit the bottom of your scope on some of your maneuvers and contaminate yourself and have to change gloves or something. When Bob is teaching and operating, he uses a 200 mm lens. When he's filming, he uses a 150. I use a 175. The light is bright enough as far as I'm concerned. I live with the 175, and that's what I routinely work with. It gives me a 7-inch working distance.

   The film speed—I photograph at sixteen frames per second. Sixteen frames per second gives you one third more exposure time than twenty-four frames. If you're going to use a 74 mm objective to get the advantage of this increased F stop, on the external scenes you'll be vignetting; you won't fill the picture. When the iris diaphragm is open wide, you get away from some of the vignetting. Once you've got the contact lens on, this vignetting and not filling the entire frame is not a problem. In order to see using the 74 mm and have the film image approximate what the surgeon is seeing, you use a 10× eyepiece. I use a 12½× eyepiece for the 137 photoadapter and a 10× eyepiece for the 74 mm. On a TV screen the 137 will fill the screen; the 74 will not unless you're working through a contact lens and are zoomed all the way up. I think that covers it pretty well.

Kasner   If a diabetic's eye is a candidate for vitrectomy, say a diabetic has blood in the vitreous for longer than a year (this is how I'm interpreting this), good light projection, retina flat by ultrasonogram, and fellow eye has good visual acuity of 20/60 or greater, would you recommend vitrectomy on the bad eye?

Okun   I wouldn't.

Douvas   I wouldn't either. If the patient insisted on it, I probably would; but I don't think the eye is harmed by letting it wait even with the blood anteriorly, so I tend to wait.

Gitter   I think it would depend a great deal on what the retina was like on that 20/60 eye, wouldn't it? I mean if it was a 20/60 eye and looked like it was going to go to light perception the next day, you'd be ready to operate on it.

Kasner   Dr. Douvas, if someone was to buy your machine, is there anything your machine cannot do?

Douvas   There're a lot of things the machine cannot do and I don't feel it has to do everything. As anyone who has participated in one of my courses knows, I use a scissors extensively. I use scissors to cut free from posterior synechiae and cut free of adherent leukoma when I can. I use a scissors to isolate cyclitic membranes that may exist, because we have to use tremendous pull to get those sometimes and I don't want to be inadvertently pulling iris or cyclitic membrane and, in turn, pull on the vitreous base. That's why I like the limbal approach on this sort of thing; and if the pupil is too small, I do a lot of it through the peripheral iridectomy that I create. The machine is an adjunct; it won't do everything.

Kasner   Dr. Peyman, what do you say about your machine?

Peyman   As a rule of thumb, any secondary membrane which I can insert a no. 52 Beaver S blade into and pass through can be removed with the vitrophage. Any membrane that's hard enough so that you cannot pass a knife through it then I would not use the vitrectomy machine. Most of those membranes are calcified or have calcified materials inside them. Any other membrane I could cut. Any nucleus that I cannot insert a knife into and any lens which I cannot make a slicing motion without dislocating I would not attempt via a pars plana approach.

Kasner Has anyone used the open sky corneal limbal incision or the corneal trephine opening?

Douvas The initial cases I did were open sky, and I had pretty good temporary results. As I recall, they also developed glaucoma postoperatively. Some became intractable, and I think this is fairly a common experience in an open sky vitrectomy in diabetic vitreous hemorrhage.

Kasner Many of us still don't have the machines. Are there still indications for the open sky technique?

Kasner After some of the things I've had with that machine, I'm ready to go back to open sky. I figure if I can rip up the eye one way, I can rip it up another.

It's true; remember that photograph I showed of Dr. Machemer working in his garage. Many times, I was thinking of calling Black & Decker and saying, "Do you want to make me some tips?" I think I can get better tips from Black & Decker than I can from present manufacturers. I would say this: for three years now, I've not done an open sky vitrectomy because I wanted to use the machine exclusively for the same indications that I had used open sky. If it weren't for the fact that the anterior segment—that means the cornea, the angle and rubbing of the iris—takes such a beating, I'd go back to open sky work in a minute. The reason is that with just your fingers, scissors, and the Weck sponges, you have exquisite control. You can go down on the retina and if you want to paint it with a little piece of Weck sponge, tickle it, you can, without hurting it. You can even dimple it with smooth forceps.

In all the years I have worked inside the retina, I think I've cracked it only twice. One was in an MVR case where I was trying very hard in an MPP situation, working on the inside of a valley, to try to pull off the membrane and the retina cracked around 5 mm away from where I was working, but very small. If I'd been working with the visc, I'd have had a hole. The other time was I once cracked the retina near the base of the vitreous. Only twice in I'd say 150 to 200 cases, I haven't counted them over the years. But in the twenty-seven cases in which I have used the visc, I've beaten my record with the other way. I'm beginning to think I may go back to the open sky for some things.

I'm not afraid of the open sky. You just have to be kind to the cornea. By that I mean if you keep it open for a couple of minutes then keep it closed for a couple of minutes. In other words, don't hold it open all the time; let it drop down. Use small sponges through the pupil, 1 × 5 mm, and you can go all the way down. If you put a ring around the eye, keep the eye elevated. The purpose of the ring is to keep the eye up so the iris falls back, keeping the angle open all the time to prevent the dvelopment of PAS.

In other words, I say to myself, "Do you think you can hurt the eye with the visc?" If I say yes, I'll go the other way. You have to think this way. Say, if you're on an archeological expedition, and sometimes going into these eyes is like that, and you can't see back there. Now what would you rather use, a pick and shovel or a ditch digger? With a pick and shovel, you can pick away. With the machine, it just grinds and grinds and sometimes the retina is behind the veils of vitreous and, before you know it, the red reflex back there is the choroid.

Kasner   Question for Dr. Shields—Why does an eye go into phthisis?

Shields   I'm not sure anybody knows the answer to that question. Apparently it is severe damage or inflammation of any type that can set it off. We all know the clinical characteristics of it.

Kasner   The reason I ask that question is, you notice that uniformly Doctors Okun, Coleman, and everybody said, "Don't wait to operate a traumatized eye." Men will get a case and they'll watch the kid 1 week, 2 weeks, and treat it with cortisone hoping something will happen. The fluffy lens will absorb. The blood inside will clear and they'll keep the case for 3 weeks, a month, and by the third month the eye is either getting rock hard or soft. They then decide maybe they'd better refer it. What is happening to this eye is that it's developing a cyclitic membrane. The cyclitic membrane, if you go into the eye, is this thick fibrinous stuff that is coating the ciliary processes. This is my idea now that when it coats the ciliary processes it literally smothers those cells. When it smothers the cells, the pump (the ciliary body) stops producing and the eye starts getting softer and dies.

   Another thing that I've noticed is you go in on an eye to clean it out with this cyclitic membrane and, as you're trying to get the last bit of cyclitic membrane off the ciliary processes, what happens? The eye up to this time is normotensive; you think you're going to do good for this eye; but by pulling on the cyclitic membrane, trying to get as close to the ciliary processes as possible, you dialyze the ciliary body. Once you've dialyzed the ciliary body, that's like producing a cyclodialysis cleft. In children that doesn't go back, and the next thing you know, 3 months later, the eye has squared off and you can't understand why it has happened.

   If you've ever had this opportunity to go in on these eyes again and you don't know what has happened but the eye is soft, you cut down on the pars plana with a sclerostomy site and you know what happens? A lot of water. The ciliary body has been dislocated. Therefore, in phthisis, two things can happen: The ciliary body epithelium can get smothered from a cyclitic membrane. The ciliary body can be dialyzed, pulled off at the scleral spur, and when that happens? The eye goes into phthisis.

Shields   That's a very interesting thought, and I think someone should look into it.

Kasner   It's not a thought, it's a fact- There was one case I recall where I thought I really had cured the case, and it subsequently went into phthisis. I was so proud of this procedure that I went back and carefully looked at the movie. It was the fourth showing when I finally saw the dialysis that I had created.

Coleman   Yes, we all agree that the ciliary body is decompensated, and David's first two reasons might be the whole story; but if we disallow the option of some possible theory of mechanism, the fluid that collects between the sclera and the ciliary body could be secondary to decompensation and infusion from the choroid.

Kasner   The point was you don't wait because the ciliary body can get smothered or else get separated; and when it's separated from the sclera, it shuts off.

Peyman   As we are starting to close the session, I'd like to thank the panelists for their fine cooperation and also thank the chairman of the symposium, Dr. Kurt Gitter, for the tremendous effort he has put into organizing this symposium. It was a very successful one.

Index